For the Love of Carbs © 2021 Emily R. Long.

All rights reserved. This book or any portion thereof may not be reproduced or used in any manner whatsoever without the express written permission of the publisher except for the use of brief quotations in a book review.

Printed in the United States of America
First Printing 2021
ISBN: 978-1-7356281-2-7
Library of Congress Control Number: 2021922144

Firefly Grace Publishing
South Burlington, VT 05403
www.EmilyRLong.com

Design by: Sarah Hubbard
Photos: Isora Lithgow (marked) and Emily Long (unmarked)
Cover: Photo by Isora Lithgow, artwork by Sarah Hubbard

For the Love of Carbs

Emily Long

Warning: Not safe for dieters.
Excessive amounts of gluten, sugar, butter,
carbohydrates, and general deliciousness.

Dedicated to Carbs.

For enjoyment, comfort, and general deliciousness.

I promise to never cut you again.

And in memory of Lisa Rowe.

I miss you every day, my friend.

You made my life more brilliant and beautiful for having had you in it.

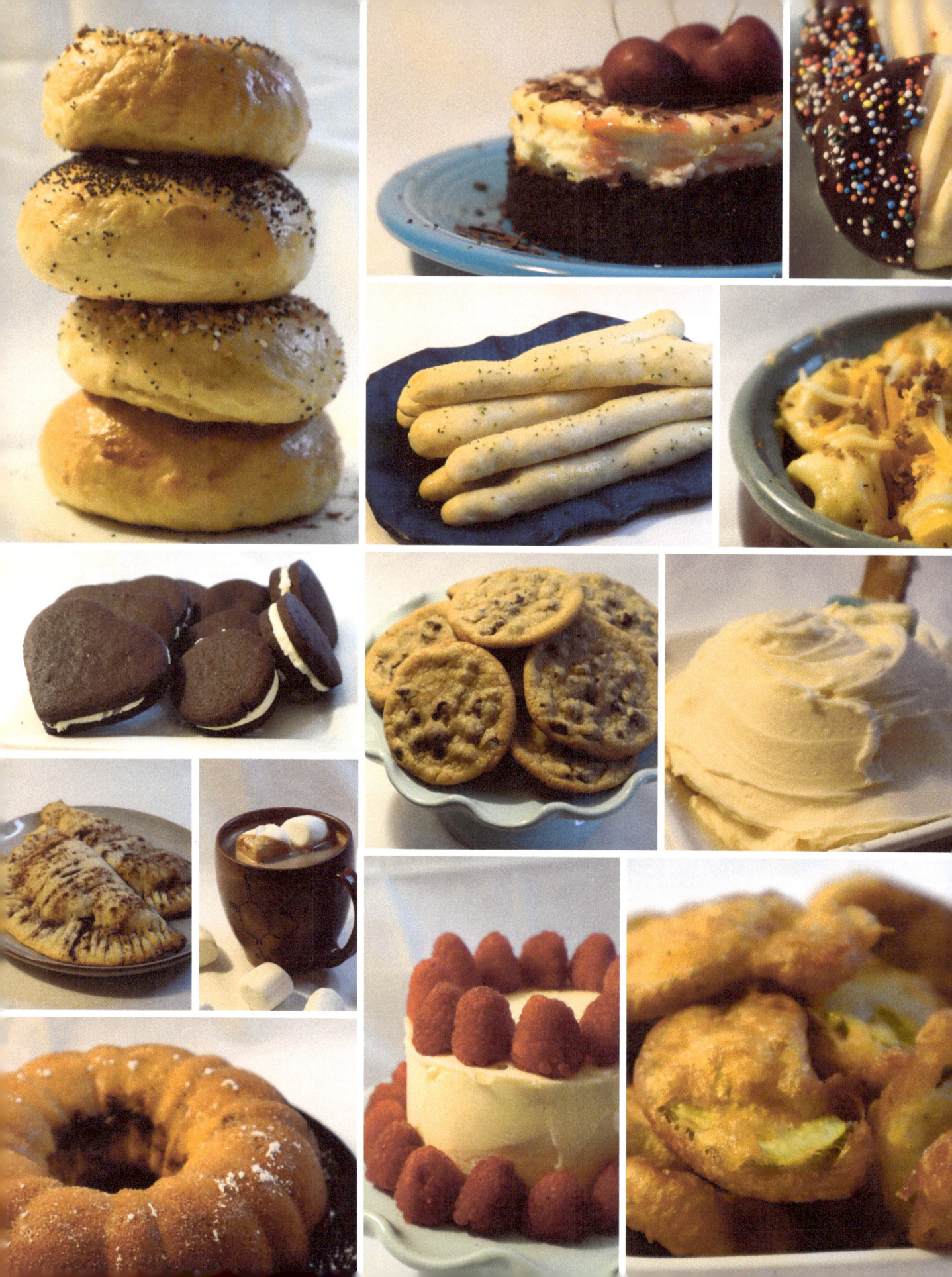

Contents

Introduction	8
Measurement Equivalents	12
Notes, Tips & Tricks	14
Recipes	16
Breakfast	18
Bread	40
Carb-licious Dinner & Sides	56
Cakes	76
Cookies	104
Just for Fun Treats	126
Pies & Tarts	144
Beverages	166
Frostings & Fillings	172
Baking Bloopers	188
Gratitude & Thank You's	191

Introduction

How 'For the Love of Carbs' was Born

The journey to this cookbook started with Mom's big silver bowl.

It's the bowl she taught me to make her amazing chocolate chip cookies in (check out page 104!) and the bowl I ate buttery salty air-popped popcorn in with Dad. I love that bowl and all the yummy and comforting childhood memories attached to it. It was my introduction to a love of baking—and a love of carbs!

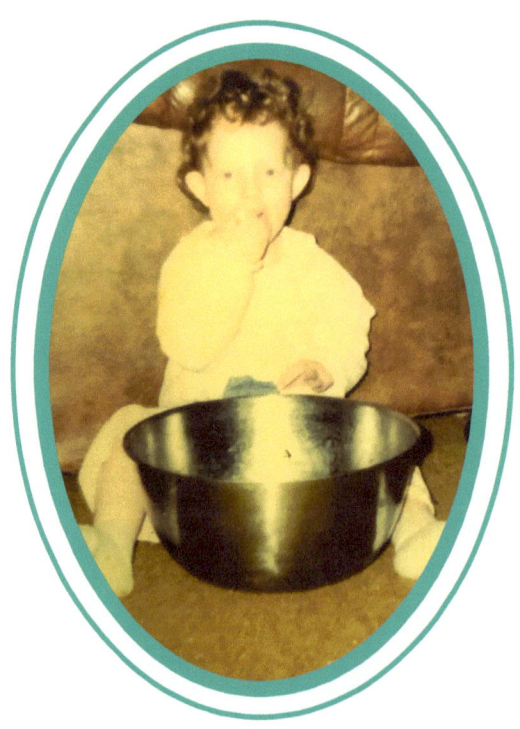

The next section of the journey came in 2013 when I randomly decided to teach myself how to make homemade bagels. Honestly, I'm not sure why I chose bagels as I wasn't much of a bagel eater up to that point. It took a few failed (and unfortunate tasting) attempts, before I achieved a decent batch. I've been refining and improving my recipe—and experimenting with fun bagel flavors—ever since. It's my favorite thing to make (and eat!).

The next section of this cookbook journey was less about baking and more about my relationship with food and body. My relationship with food has always been... we'll say fraught with angst and pain. I had and have sensory and taste aversions, which in my childhood and early adulthood made food choices limited and difficult—and had painful social impacts. I always felt something was wrong with me because I gravitated toward starchy carbs, fruits, and simple, uncomplicated foods. I have never eaten meat, vegetables were a struggle for many, many years (so bitter!), and mixing too many flavors or strong spices together was intolerable. Eating out or eating in social situations was difficult, full of anxiety, and emotionally painful.

As a result, my relationship with food (and in connection, with my body) was full of shame, self-criticism and self-hate. Until 2018 that is, when I found the anti-diet and Health at Every Size (HAES) community. I learned that I could just be me—as "weird" and different and fat-bodied and carb-loving as I was—and it was ok. My body was my body. My eating was my eating. And I learned that so many of the things that we're taught about food and body and health and nutrition are deeply rooted in racism, anti-fat bias, and are, well, fucked up. So very fucked up.

> I learned that I could just be me—as "weird" and different and fat-bodied and carb-loving as I was—and it was ok.

It was like being set free. I could finally eat and enjoy food. I could eat what I ate and not worry about it. I could eat and not spend hours every day thinking about food or spending so much time and mental energy counting calories or "burning it off" or obsessing if I was "doing it right or eating too much or too little of XYZ." Food became fun again. It became joy and comfort. It became uncomplicated and, most importantly, emotionally and morally neutral.

Then came 2020 and the stress of being a mental health therapist during the coronavirus pandemic. Days that became weeks that became months and years of staying home and, as I was single and living alone, being very isolated. There was also the intense worry about loved ones who were vulnerable, grief for loved ones who died of Covid, and trying to support clients through this global trauma while also navigating it myself.

I coped by baking. A lot of baking. *So much baking.*

I tried new recipes by other people. Then I experimented with adapting recipes. Then I started making my own. My grocery list became filled with flour, salt, butter, milk, sugar, cornstarch, baking chocolate, vanilla (*always* vanilla!), herbs, sprinkles, and all the other things that make delicious carb based recipes.

When my freezer got full and I couldn't eat it all by myself, I left goody packages on the porches of friends, mailed boxes of cookies to friends around the country, and gave baked goods as gifts. Friends started asking for recipes and requesting tips and tricks.

Sometime around late summer or early fall 2020, I had the idea—"well, why not turn all these recipes into a cookbook?" I had published 8 previous books on pregnancy and infant loss and had been wanting to shift to less heavy and emotionally tender writing. As baking had always been a part of my personal grieving process, expanding my area of work in that direction and writing a cookbook seemed a perfect pivot.

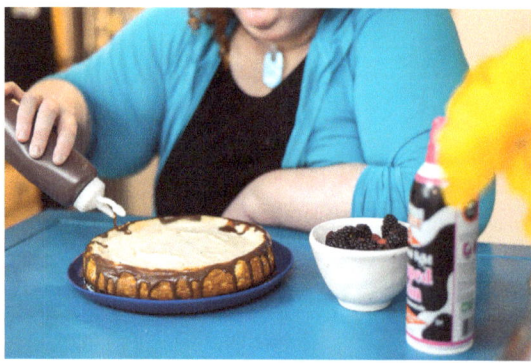

Photos by Tsora Lithgow

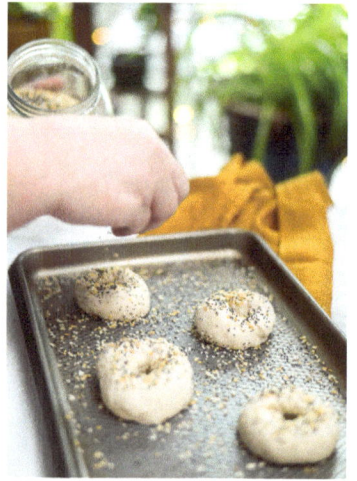

That's how "For the Love of Carbs" was born—out of childhood, fun experimentation, healing, and surviving a life-altering pandemic. These are the things I poured into these recipes and this book—love and fun and play and deep healing and pleasure and comfort and deliciousness and *life*.

I hope you experience all of that as you try out these recipes.

Carbs and I hope that you enjoy and savor every delicious bite.

In gratitude and love,

Emily

P.S. This book is unintentionally vegetarian. Solely because I happen to be a life-long vegetarian (see: sensory food aversions) and I just don't cook or bake with meat. And, yes, that includes chicken or fish as those are also meat. (My fellow vegetarians will understand the need to specify that!) However, meat could easily be added to many of these recipes for the meat-eaters among you—I just can't tell you how to cook it!

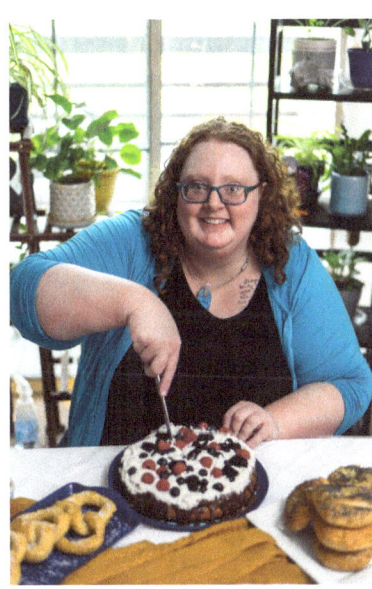
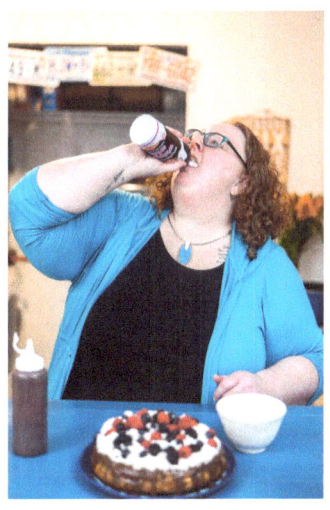

Photos by Tiara Lithgow

Measurement Equivalents

Measurement Equivalents

1 tablespoon = 3 teaspoons

2 tablespoons = 1 liquid oz

4 tablespoons = ¼ cup

5 ⅓ tablespoons = ⅓ cup

8 tablespoons = ½ cup

1 egg = 4 tablespoons liquid

4-5 eggs = 1 cup

7-9 egg whites = 1 cup

12-14 egg yolks = 1 cup

1 cup uncooked rice = 3 cups cooked

1 cup uncooked pasta = 2 to 2 ¼ cups cooked

6 oz chocolate chips = 1 cup

3 ⅓ tablespoon cocoa + ½ tablespoon butter = 1 oz chocolate

Substitutions

1 cup buttermilk = 1 tablespoon white vinegar or lemon juice + enough milk to make 1 cup, and let sit for 5 minutes
OR: 1 cup plain yogurt

1 cup heavy cream = 1/3 cup butter + 3/4 cup milk

1 tablespoon cornstarch (for thickening) = 2 tablespoons flour

1 cup cake flour = 7/8 cup flour + 2 tablespoons of cornstarch and sift well

1 cup corn syrup = 1 cup sugar + 1/4 cup water (or other liquid recipe calls for)

1 tsp baking powder = 1/4 tsp baking soda + 1/2 tsp cream of tarter

1 cup honey = 1 1/4 cup granulated sugar + 1/4 cup water

1 small clove garlic = 1 1/8 tsp garlic powder

1/2 tsp white vinegar = 1 tsp lemon juice

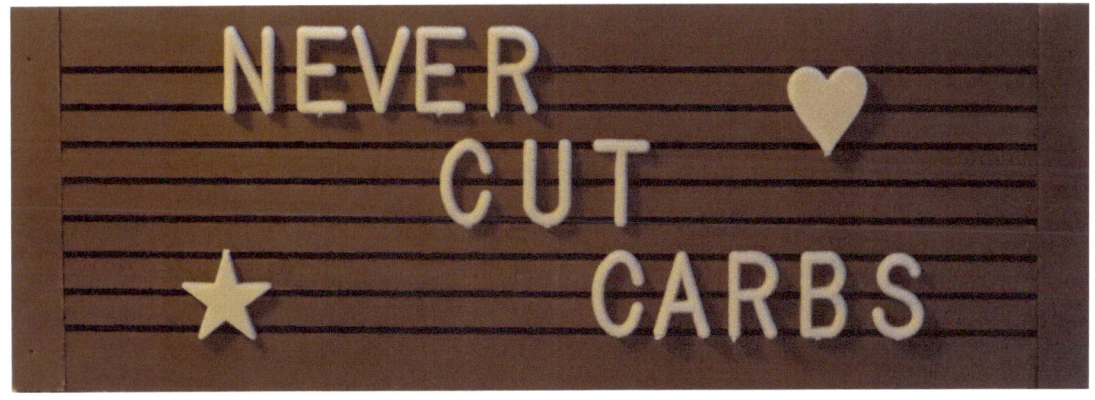

Notes, Tips & Tricks

General Notes to Know

- Assume all-purpose flour unless otherwise specified
- Assume sugar means granulated sugar unless otherwise specified
- All temperatures are in Fahrenheit
- tbsp = tablespoon
- tsp = teaspoon

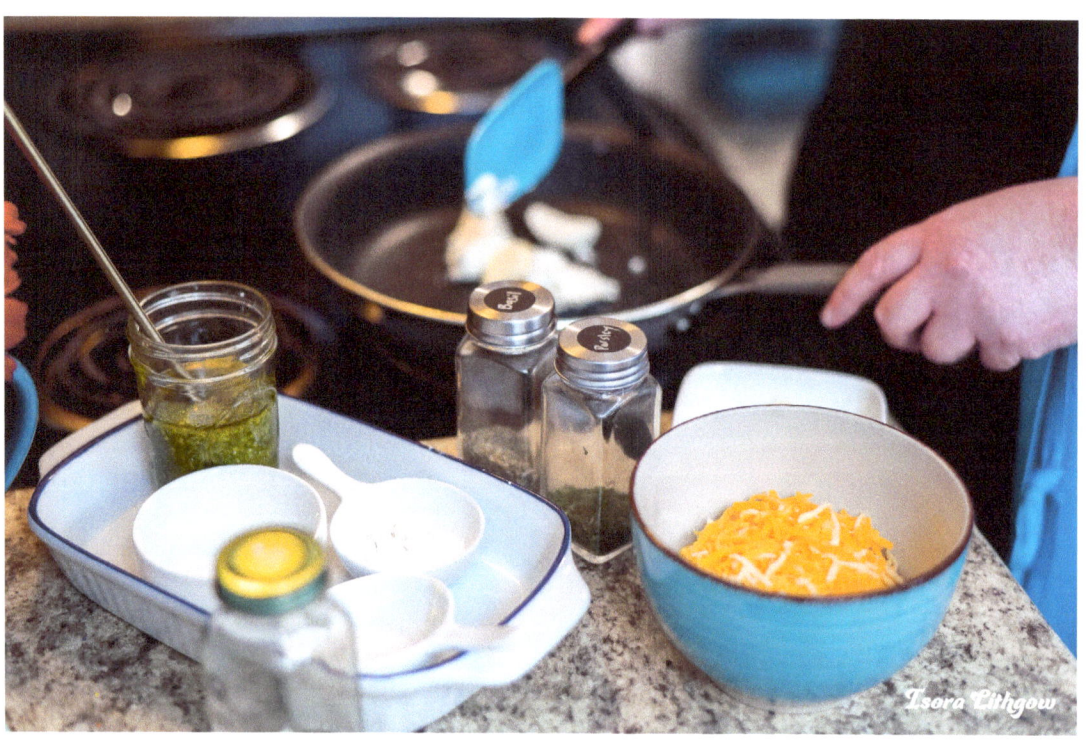

Tips & Tricks

- Always scrape the sides of bowl while mixing at least 1-3 times to ensure fully incorporating all ingredients.

- Roll cookie doughs out between two pieces of parchment paper or wax paper for ease and to reduce sticking.

- Bread proofing is complete when dent remains when poked but doesn't collapse in.

- Always cream butter and sugar a minute longer than you think you should.

- Remove cookies from oven just before they look done!

- To add sugar or granulated sprinkles to cookies or cakes, use a salt shaker for more even dusting! A shaker can also be used for dusting flour when hand kneading bread or rolling out cookie dough.

- When melting chocolate, grease the pan first, it'll help prevent sticking.

- Grease the measuring spoon or cup before measuring out honey, molasses, or other sticky ingredients.

- Instead of wasting eggs for egg washes, keep a container of liquid egg whites to use instead!

- When it says room temperature for ingredients—use room temperature ingredients!!

- You can grate cold butter for quicker softened butter, or place butter under an upside down hot bowl or pan for a minute.

- To quickly bring eggs to room temperature, place them in warm water for 3-5 minutes.

Recipes

Breakfast	12
Bread	40
Carb-licious Dinners & Sides	56
Cakes	76

Photo by Isora Lithgow

Cookies	**104**
Just for Fun Treats	**126**
Pies & Tarts	**144**
Beverages	**166**
Frostings & Fillings	**172**

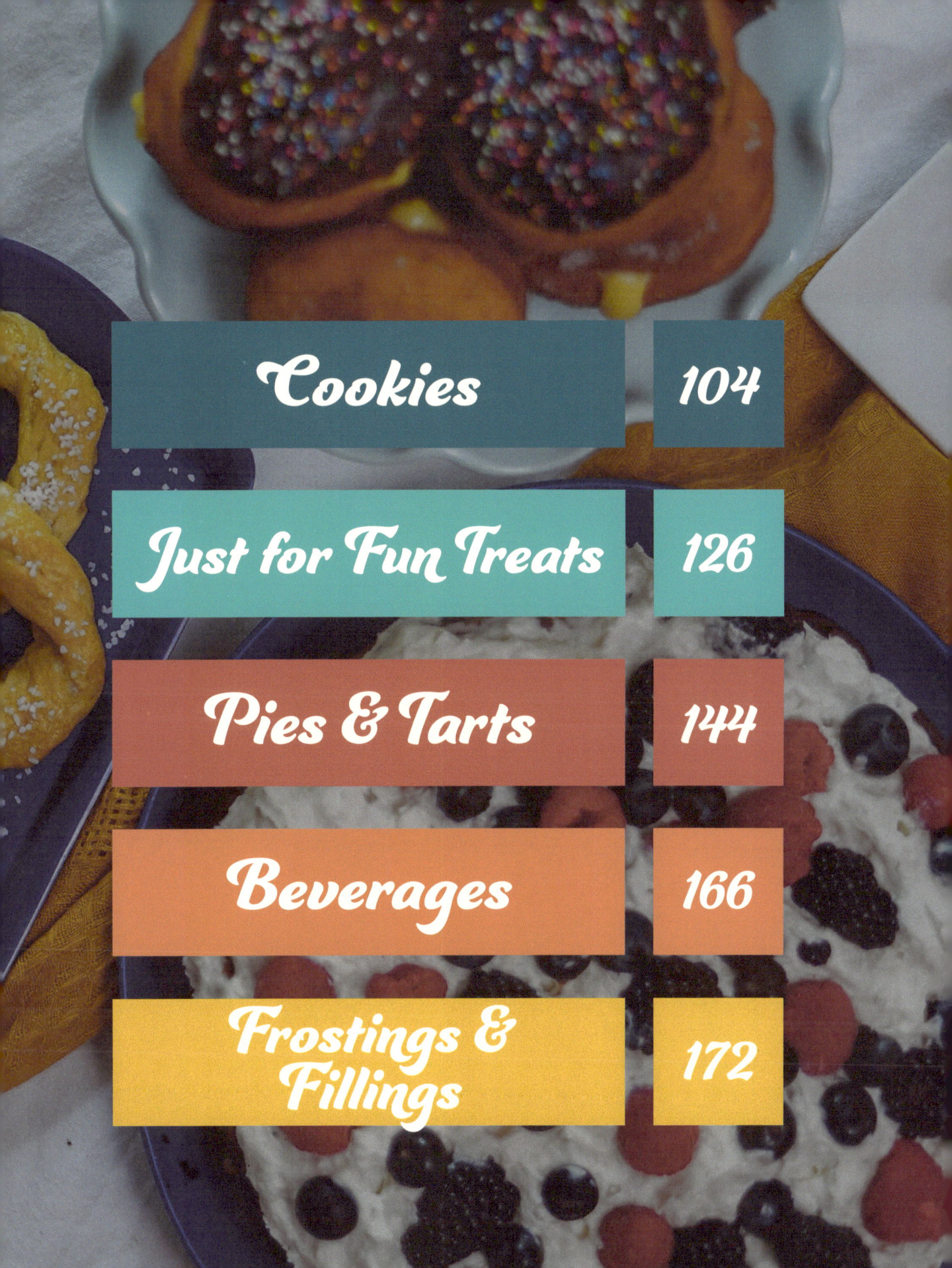

Emily's Bagels

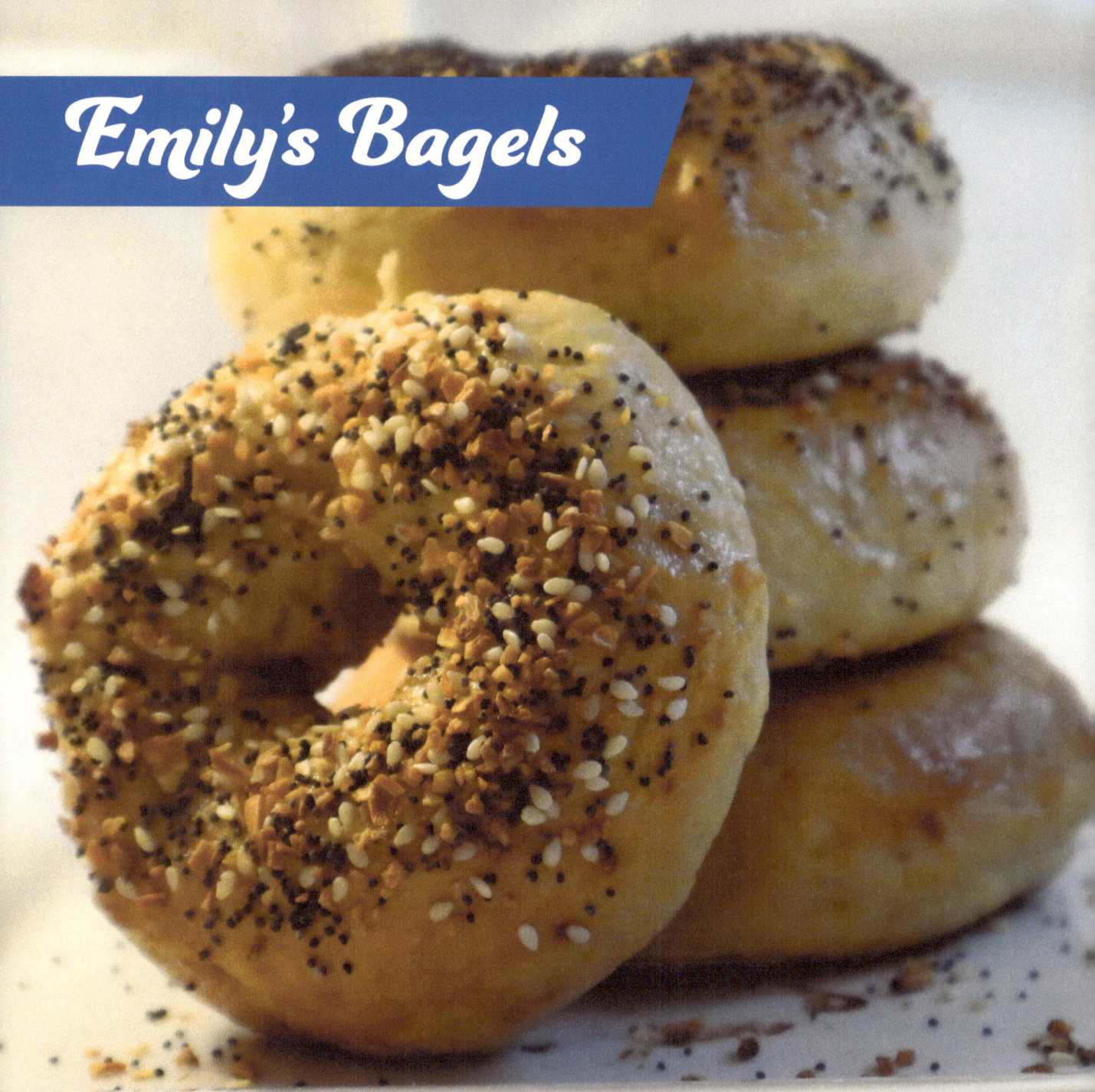

I love to bake all the things, but these bagels are my specialty—and my favorite. Soft but chewy, every bite is sheer joy. These beauties started me on this journey of baking experimentation and nothing is more fun than trying creative additions and toppings. They are a process to make—though not nearly as hard as one might believe—and I find the process of kneading, shaping, and forming them to be meditative. Nothing beats a fresh from the oven, warm bagel, but these also freeze well and can easily be made ahead or saved for future events. Word of caution, however, these will ruin you for store-bought bagels—and even most bagel shop bagels. They're just that good.

Serving:
10-12 bagels

Prep Time:
1 hour, 40 minutes

Bake Time:
20 minutes

Ingredients

- 1 ½ cups warm (not hot) water
- 2 tsp dry active yeast
- 1 ½ tbsp sugar
- 2 tsp salt
- 3 ½ cups bread flour
- 2 tbsp molasses
- Optional: egg wash and toppings or mix-in ingredients of choice (see suggestions below)

Directions

1. Mix warm water with yeast and sugar in a small bowl. Let sit for about 5 minutes until foamy.
2. Add flour and salt to the mixing bowl and whisk together.
3. Add yeast water to flour and salt.
4. With a dough hook, mix on medium speed until combined. (If adding ingredients to the dough, add now) continue to knead dough until tacky and smooth.
5. Cover bowl and set aside to rise for about 1 hour until doubled in size.
6. Once risen, set a large pot of water with molasses on the stove to boil and preheat the oven to 425°F.
7. Divide dough into small balls, flatten slightly, and use your thumb to shape into traditional bagel shapes. Set on a baking sheet to rest.
8. Once the pot is boiling, place several pieces (depending on size of pot, 2-4 at a time) of shaped dough into boiling water for 1-2 minutes, flipping about halfway through.
9. Scoop out and return to the baking sheet. Repeat until all bagels have been boiled.
10. If adding toppings, brush with egg wash and sprinkle with toppings of choice.
11. Bake for 18-20 minutes at 425°F or until golden brown.
12. Remove from the oven and enjoy!

Note:

These freeze well—for quick use, slice before freezing and pop into toaster straight from the freezer.

Will keep in an airtight container on the counter for 2-3 days, best to freeze if longer than this to prevent mold.

Emily's Bagels
continued

Variations

Toppings:

- Everything Bagel Seasoning
- Pretzel salt
- Cinnamon sugar
- Poppy seeds
- Sesame Seeds

Mix-Ins:

- Herbs
- Chocolate chips or mini M&Ms
- Dried raspberries and chocolate chips
- Peanut butter chips and chocolate chips
- Lime zest (add pretzel salt topping)
- Lemon zest and dried blueberries
- Pesto
- Dried apples and cinnamon
- Dried apples and peanut butter chips
- Garlic and Parmesan
- Garlic
- Dried cranberry and pumpkin seed
- Lemon zest (poppy seed topping)
- And more! Be creative :)

Double Recipe (20-22 bagels)

- 3 cups warm (not hot) water
- 4 tsp dry active yeast
- 3 tbsp sugar
- 4 tsp salt
- 7 cups bread flour

Single Serve (5-6 bagels)

- 1 cup + ½ tbsp warm water
- 1 ½ tsp dry active yeast
- 1 tbsp sugar
- 1 ½ tsp salt
- 2 ⅓ cups bread flour

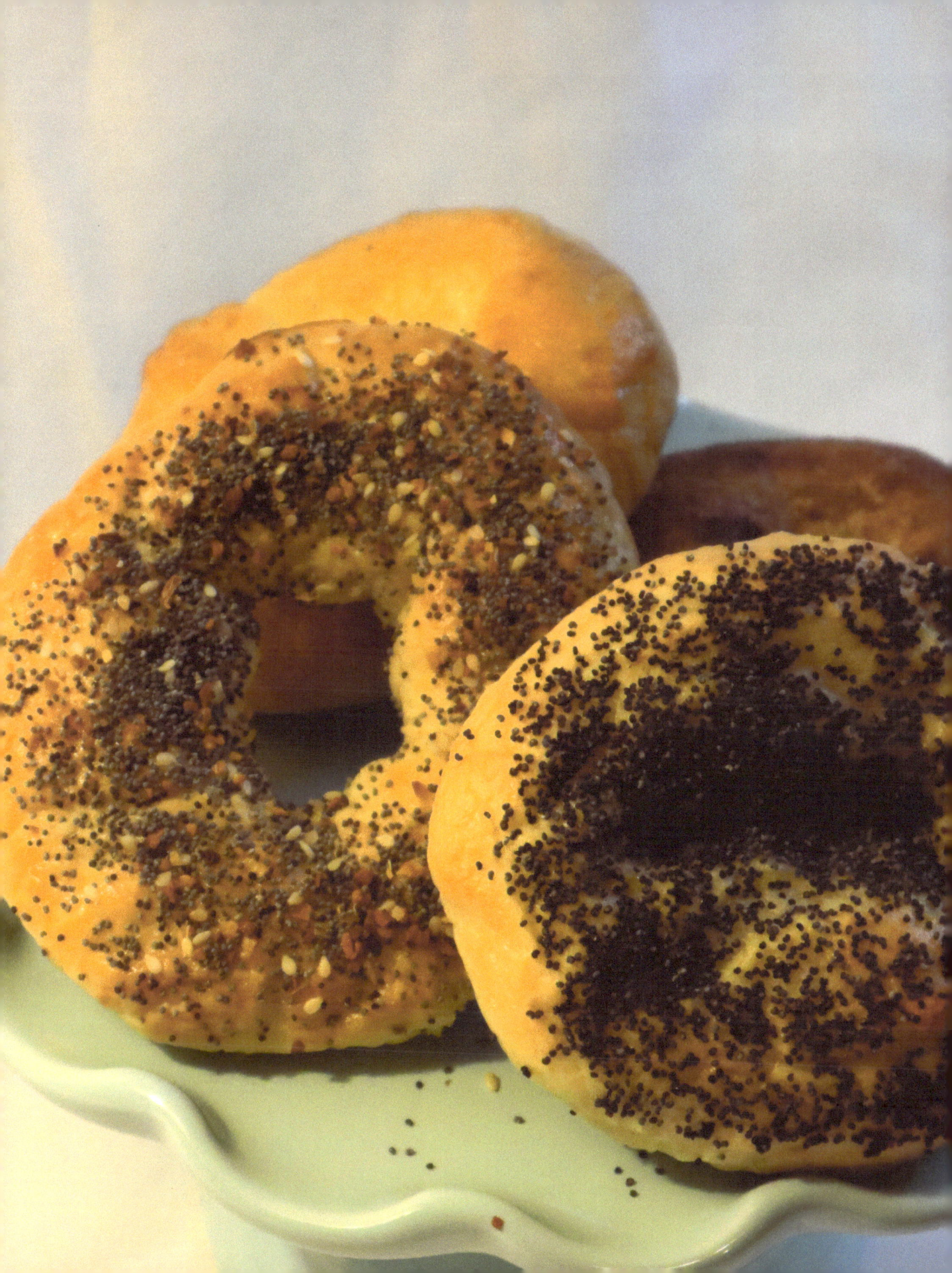

Popovers

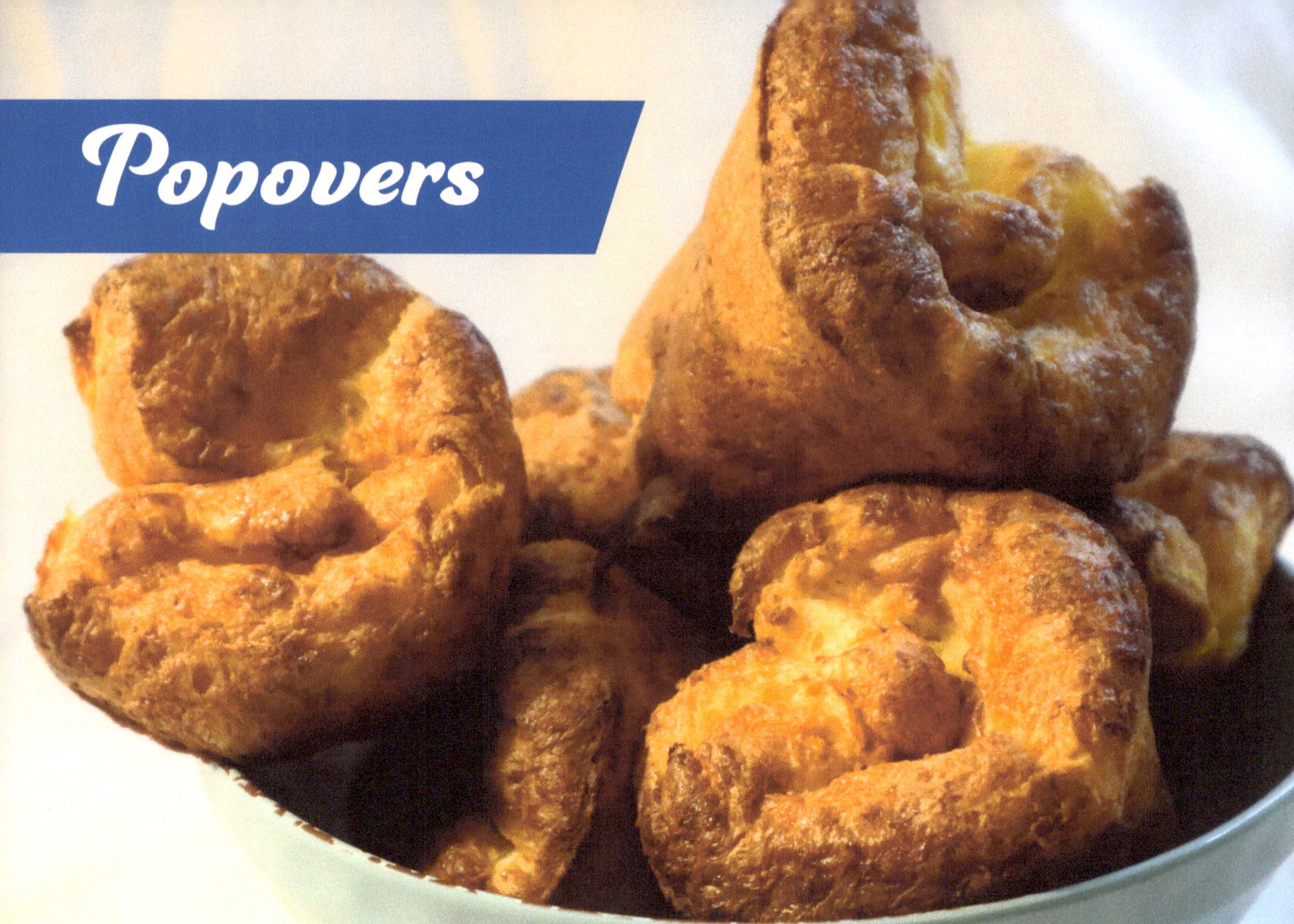

It's like a pancake crossed with an egg-y croissant. Or a Dutch baby combined with a muffin. It's carb-perfection shaped like a muffin but hollow, just waiting to be stuffed with jam or cheese or eggs or other deliciousness. Okay, so it's hard to explain. Let's just say it's absolutely worth waiting for room temperature ingredients and is an absolute must try. Trust me.

Serving:
6 popovers

Prep Time:
35 minutes

Bake Time:
30-35 minutes

Ingredients

- 3 large eggs, room temp
- 1 cup + 2 tbsp milk, room temp
- 1 cup flour
- ½ tsp salt
- 1½ tbsp melted butter + 1 tbsp for pan

Note:
Room temperature ingredients are very important to get the best "pop" or rise while baking. Don't skip this step!

Directions

1. Spoon flour into measuring cup (or shift through fine mesh strainer).
2. Whisk flour and salt together.
3. Add room temperature milk, eggs, and melted butter and whisk until smooth. Batter should be fairly thin and run off whisk.
4. Let batter rest for 15-30 minutes while preheating the oven to 450°F, heat the popover pan (on top of a baking sheet) until hot.
5. Remove popover pan from oven.
6. Brush popover cups generously with remaining melted butter.
7. Fill cups about half full with batter (try to do in one pour, don't top off or won't rise as well).
8. Return to oven.
9. Bake at 450°F for 15 minutes; reduce heat to 375°F, bake for 15 minutes until deep golden brown.
   Note: do NOT open the oven for the first 30 minutes of bake time.
10. When golden brown, remove from the oven, poke hole in each popover & take popovers from the pan immediately.
11. Enjoy!

Variations

- Sprinkle teaspoon of mini chocolate chips into batter just before baking (don't mix).
- Add sprinkle of shredded cheese onto batter just before baking (again, don't mix).
- Brush with butter and roll in cinnamon sugar after baking.
- Brush with butter and roll in garlic salt and grated Parmesan cheese after baking.
- Fill with peanut butter, jam, scrambled eggs, shredded cheese, etc. after baking.

Note:

Can use a large 6 cup muffin pan instead of a popover pan.

Can also make mini versions using a 12 cup muffin pan.

Double Recipe (12 popovers)

- 6 large eggs, room temp
- 2 ¼ cups milk, room temp
- 2 cups flour
- 1 tsp salt
- 3 tbsp melted butter + 2 tbsp for pan

Single Serve (3 popovers)

- 2 medium eggs, room temp
- ½ cup + 1 tbsp milk, room temp
- ½ cup flour
- ¼ tsp. salt
- ¾ tbsp melted butter + ½ tbsp for pan

Cinnamon Rolls

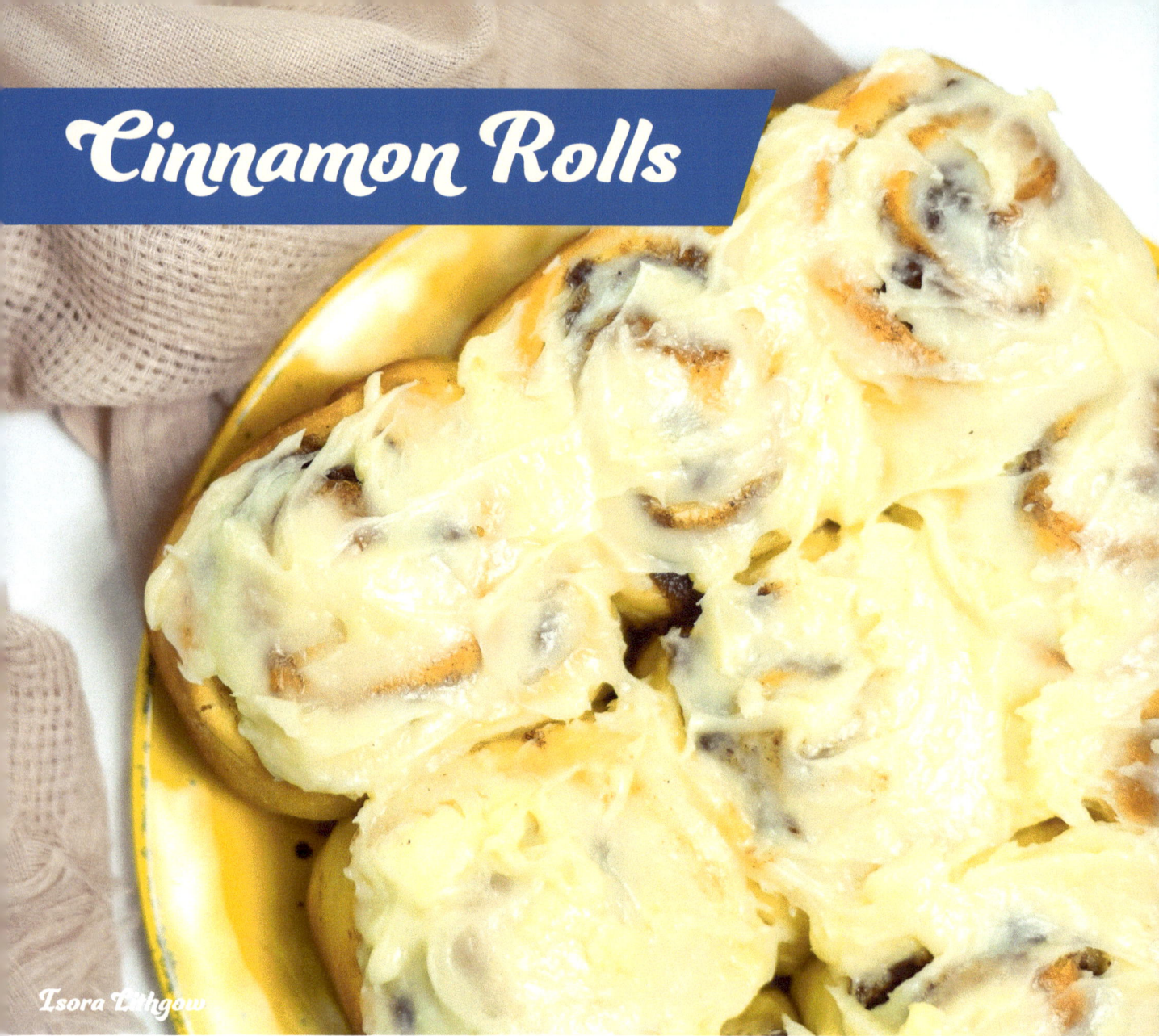

Isora Lithgow

It took me years to learn to make good cinnamon rolls. For whatever reason, I just never could get them to rise properly for the soft, tender bite I wanted. After years of tossed batches, I finally found my perfect roll of cinnamon delicious—with a twist of cream cheese. Soft and sweet with a subtle tang of cream cheese—absolutely worth all the failed attempts over the years. Cinnamon perfection.

Serving:
10-12 rolls

Prep Time:
3 hours

Bake Time:
20-30 minutes

Ingredients

Tangzhong
- ½ cup milk
- 3 tbsp bread flour

Dough
- ¾ cup milk
- 3 ½ cups bread flour
- 2 ¼ tsp instant yeast
- 2 tbsp sugar
- ¼ tsp salt
- 3 large eggs
- 1 ½ tsp vanilla
- 1 stick (½ cup) melted butter

Filling
- 1 tbsp melted butter
- ½ cup packed brown sugar
- 3-4 tsp cinnamon
- ½ tsp nutmeg
- 2 tbsp bread flour
- Pinch of salt
- 8 oz cream cheese, softened

Icing
- 1 ½ tbsp melted butter
- 5 tbsp cream cheese, softened
- 1 tsp vanilla
- Pinch of salt
- 1 ½ cups sifted powdered sugar
- 1 to 2 tbsp milk (enough to thin to desired consistency)

Breakfast

Directions

Tangzhong
- Combine milk and flour in saucepan and whisk until lump-free.
- Place saucepan over medium heat and cook, mixing regularly, until thickened and paste-like, leaving spoon/spatula lines at bottom of pan. (Approximately 1-3 minutes.)
- Remove from heat and transfer to large mixing bowl (whatever you plan to mix remaining ingredients in).

> **Note:** Can skip the tangzhong, but it helps keep rolls softer for longer.

Dough
1. Add all ingredients, starting with milk (heat from tangzhong will help warm cold milk) and mix to bring dough together.
2. Knead dough until smooth, elastic, and tacky (not sticky). Approximately 10-15 minutes.
3. Shape into a ball, place in a lightly oiled bowl, cover with plastic wrap and let sit for about 1 hour until puffy/doubled in size.

Filling
4. Add melted butter to a medium bowl, add brown sugar, cinnamon, nutmeg, flour, and pinch of salt. Mix until the texture of wet sand.
5. Lightly grease or line baking sheet. Transfer dough to lightly greased work surface and press into about 10x16 rectangle.

Cinnamon Rolls
continued

6. Spread softened cream cheese over dough, leaving about a ½ in strip along one long side.
7. Sprinkle filling over the cream cheese dough
8. Begin to roll into a tight log starting with filling the covered side and pinch together with ½-inch strips of bare dough.
9. Lightly score log into equal 1 ½ – 2-inch pieces.
10. Cut with a sharp knife or dental floss and place onto the prepared baking sheet.
11. Cover and let rise for 20-30 minutes.
12. Preheat the oven to 350°F. Bake for 20-30 minutes or until golden brown. (Less time for softer rolls, more for firmer.)

Icing

13. Combine icing ingredients in a medium bowl, mixing until smooth. Add milk slowly until it achieves desired consistency.

Variations

- Substitute buttermilk for milk in icing for slightly tangier flavor.
- For non-cream cheese icing, simply omit cream cheese and mix remaining ingredients.

Note:

Can also skip the cream cheese spread for filling but it adds a lovely softness and mild cream cheese tang that is amazing!

If saving for later, wait to add icing until serving. Wrap tightly and freeze.

Double Recipe (20-24 rolls)

Tangzhong
- ½ cup milk
- 3 tbsp bread flour

Dough
- 1 ½ cups milk
- 7 cups bread flour
- 4 ½ tsp instant yeast
- 4 tbsp sugar
- ½ tsp salt
- 6 large eggs
- 3 tsp vanilla
- 2 stick (1 cup) melted butter

Filling
- 2 tbsp melted butter
- 1 cup packed brown sugar
- 2 tbsp cinnamon
- 1 tsp nutmeg
- 4 tbsp bread flour
- ¼ tsp salt
- 16 oz cream cheese, softened

Icing
- 3 tbsp melted butter
- 10 tbsp cream cheese, softened
- 2 tsp vanilla
- ¼ tsp salt
- 3 cups sifted powdered sugar
- 2 to 4 tbsp milk (enough to thin to desired consistency)

Single Serve (6 rolls)

Tangzhong
- ¼ cup milk
- 1 ½ tbsp bread flour

Dough
- ¼ cup + 2 tbsp milk
- 1 ¾ cups bread flour
- 1 ⅛ tsp instant yeast
- 1 tbsp sugar
- ⅛ tsp salt
- 1 ½ large eggs
- ¾ tsp vanilla
- ½ stick (¼ cup) melted butter

Filling
- ½ tbsp melted butter
- ¼ cup packed brown sugar
- 2-3 tsp cinnamon
- ¼ tsp nutmeg
- 1 tbsp bread flour
- Pinch of salt
- 4 oz cream cheese, softened

Icing
- ¾ tbsp melted butter
- 2-3 tbsp cream cheese, softened
- ½ tsp vanilla
- Pinch of salt
- ¾ cup sifted powdered sugar
- ½ to 1 tbsp milk (enough to thin to desired consistency)

Breakfast

Waffles

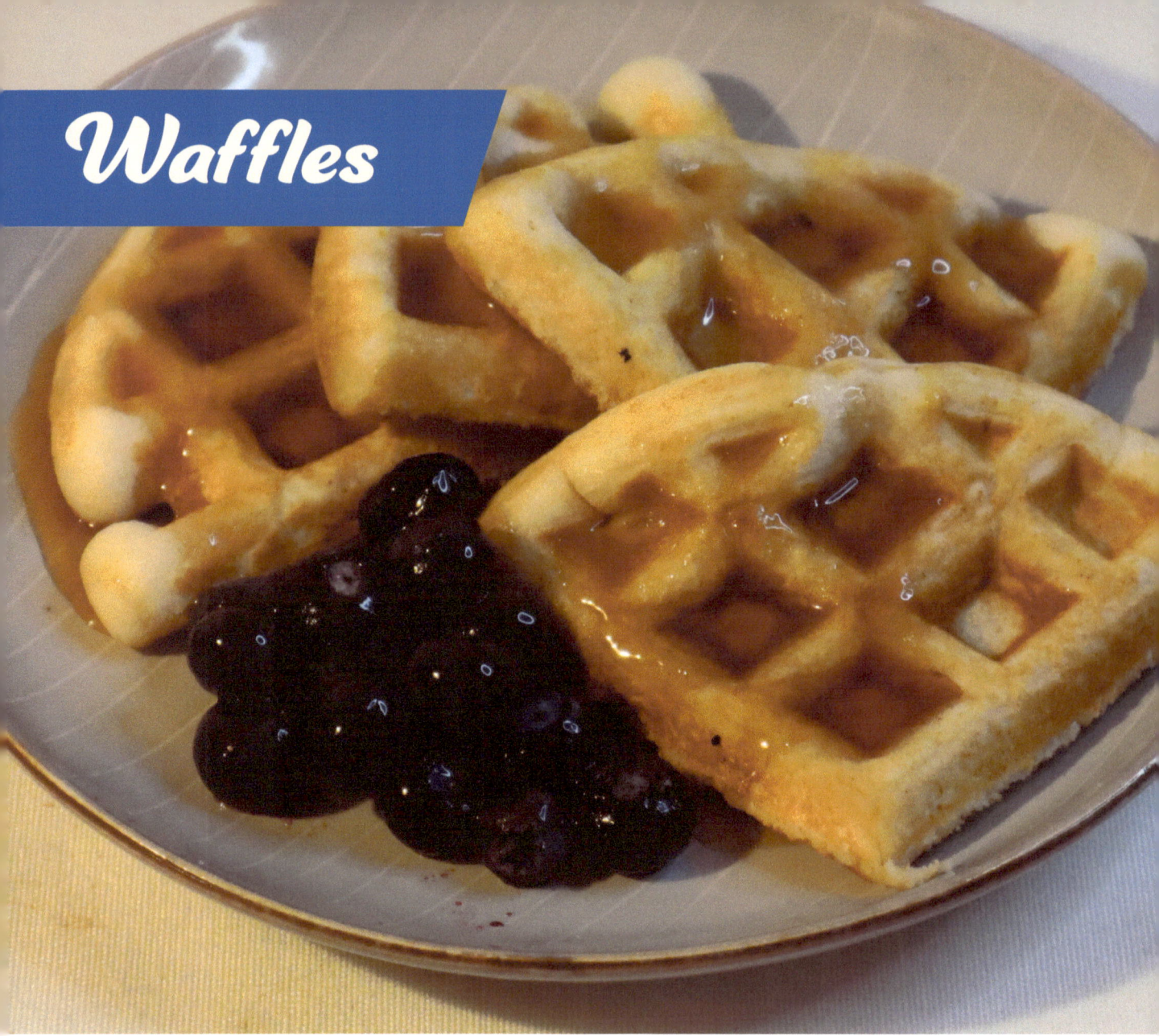

Waffles make me think of slow weekend mornings, breakfast out laughing with friends, and hotel trips as a kid, so excited to make a waffle in the Belgian waffle machine. Cook them until they're golden brown, slightly crisp on the outside and chewy inside, and feast on them smothered in melted butter, berries or chocolate chips, or powdered sugar. Add whipped cream if you are feeling extra indulgent—or stick with the classic maple syrup. 100% worth the investment in a quality waffle iron!

Serving:
3-5 waffles (depending on waffle iron)

Prep Time:
10 minutes

Bake Time:
10 minutes

Ingredients

- 1 cup + 2 tbsp flour
- ½ tbsp baking powder
- 1 ½ tbsp sugar
- ¼ tsp salt
- ½ tsp cinnamon
- 1 large egg, separated
- ¼ cup vegetable oil
- 1 cup milk
- 1 tsp vanilla

Directions

1. Preheat waffle iron and coat with oil or cooking spray.
2. In a large bowl, whisk together the flour, baking powder, sugar, salt and cinnamon.
3. Separate egg yolk and egg white.
4. Beat egg white until stiff peaks form. (I highly recommend an electric whisk!)
5. Add egg yolk, vegetable oil, milk, and vanilla to dry ingredients and mix.
6. Fold in egg whites.
7. Pour batter into hot waffle iron.
8. Serve hot with butter, syrup, and favorite toppings.
9. Enjoy!

Variations

- Add chocolate chips to batter.
- Add favorite fruits to batter.
- Top with peanut butter or fresh fruit.
- Top with jam.
- Dust with powdered sugar.
- Pile on the whipped cream.

Double Recipe (6-8 waffles)

- 2 ¼ cups flour
- 1 tbsp baking powder
- 3 tbsp sugar
- ½ tsp salt
- 1 tsp cinnamon
- 2 large eggs, separated
- ½ cup vegetable oil
- 2 cups milk
- 2 tsp vanilla

Single Serve (1-2 waffles)

- ½ cup + 1 tbsp flour
- ¼ tbsp baking powder
- ¾ tbsp sugar
- ⅛ tsp salt
- ¼ tsp cinnamon
- 1 large egg, separated
- 2 tbsp vegetable oil
- ½ cup milk
- ½ tsp vanilla

Breakfast

Cream Cheese Bagel Bombs

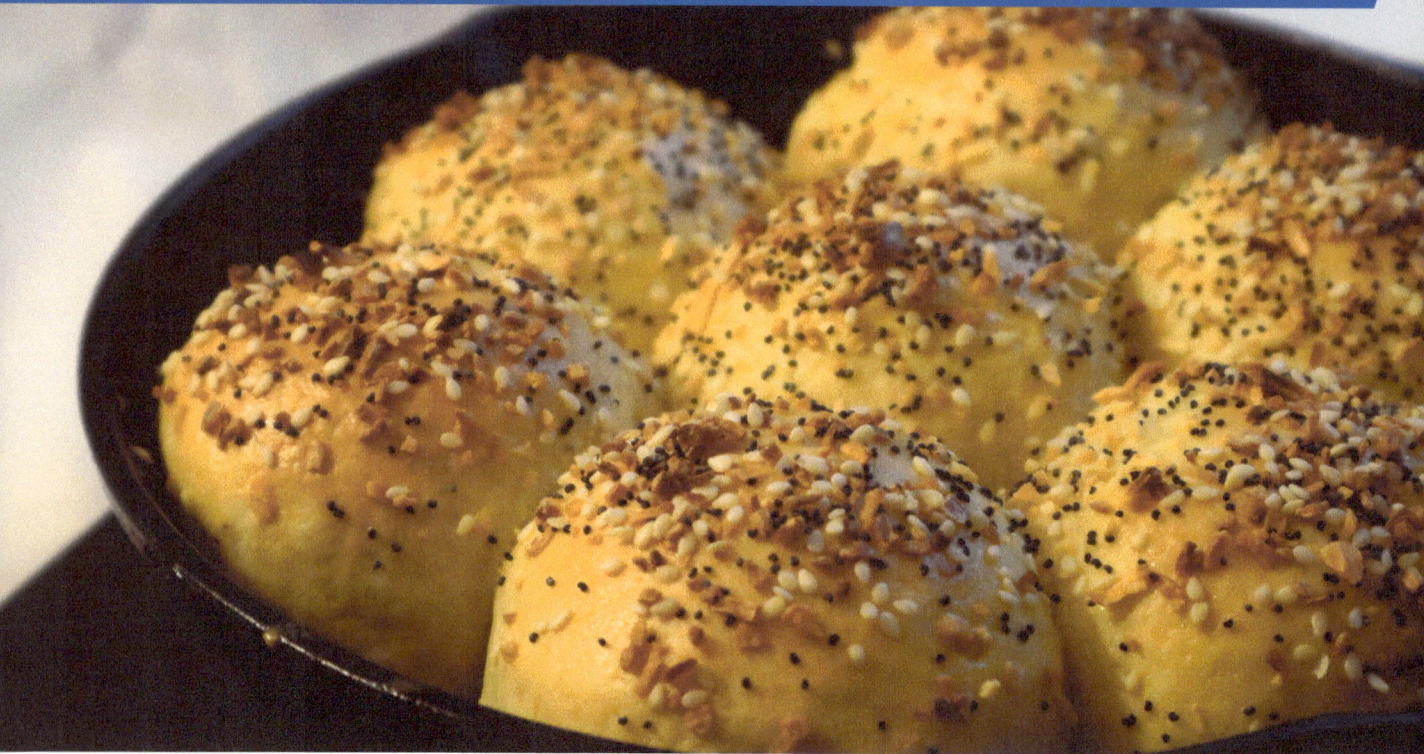

Classic bagels will always be my favorite, but these melty cream cheese filled bites are a tough competitor! Chewy bagel wrapped around warm, soft cream cheese is a mouthful of bliss. These bite-sized nuggets are best eaten warm, (but not hot because that melted cream cheese can burn!) fresh from the pan. Not that leftovers will be an issue—it's doubtful you'll be able to resist finishing off these delightful bites.

Serving:
12 bagel bombs

Prep Time:
1 hour, 10 minutes

Bake Time:
15-18 minutes

Ingredients

- 1 cup + ½ tbsp warm water
- 1 ½ tsp dry active yeast
- 1 tbsp sugar
- 2 ⅓ cups bread flour
- 1 ½ tsp salt
- 8 oz cream cheese, cubed into 12 pieces.

Directions

1. Mix water with yeast and sugar in a small bowl. Let sit for about 5 minutes until foamy.
2. Add flour and salt to the mixing bowl and mix.
3. Add yeast water to flour and salt.
4. With a dough hook, mix on medium speed until combined. Continue to knead dough until tacky and smooth.
5. Cover bowl and set aside to rise for about 1 hour until doubled in size.
6. Once risen, set a large pot of water on the stove to boil and preheat the oven to 425°F.
7. Divide dough into 12 small balls. Flatten slightly, add a cube of cream cheese and wrap dough around it. Roll in hands to seal.
8. Once the pot is boiling, place several dough balls into boiling water for 1-2 minutes, flipping about halfway through.
9. Scoop out and arrange in a cast iron pan. Repeat until all have been boiled.
10. If adding toppings, brush with egg wash and sprinkle with toppings of choice.
11. Bake in a cast iron pan in the oven for 15-20 minutes at 425°F or until golden brown.
12. Remove from the oven, let cool for 10-15 minutes, and enjoy!

Variations

Toppings:
- Everything Bagel Seasoning
- Pretzel salt
- Cinnamon sugar
- Poppy seeds
- Sesame Seeds

Flavored Cream Cheese Options:
- Herbs
- Cinnamon
- Pesto
- Avocado and lime

Note:
Cream cheese will be very hot so be cautious!

Can use a baking sheet or Dutch oven if you don't have a cast iron pan.

Best eaten fresh and warm!

Double Recipe
(24 bagel bombs)

- 2 cups + 1 tbsp warm water
- 3 tsp dry active yeast
- 2 tbsp sugar
- 4 2/3 cup bread flour
- 3 tsp salt
- 16 oz cream cheese, cubed into 24 pieces

Single Serve
(6 bagel bombs)

- ½ cup + 1 tsp warm water
- ¾ tsp dry active yeast
- ½ tbsp sugar
- 1 cup + 2 ½ tbsp bread flour
- ¾ tsp salt
- 4 oz cream cheese, cubed into 6 pieces

Dutch Baby (German Pancake)

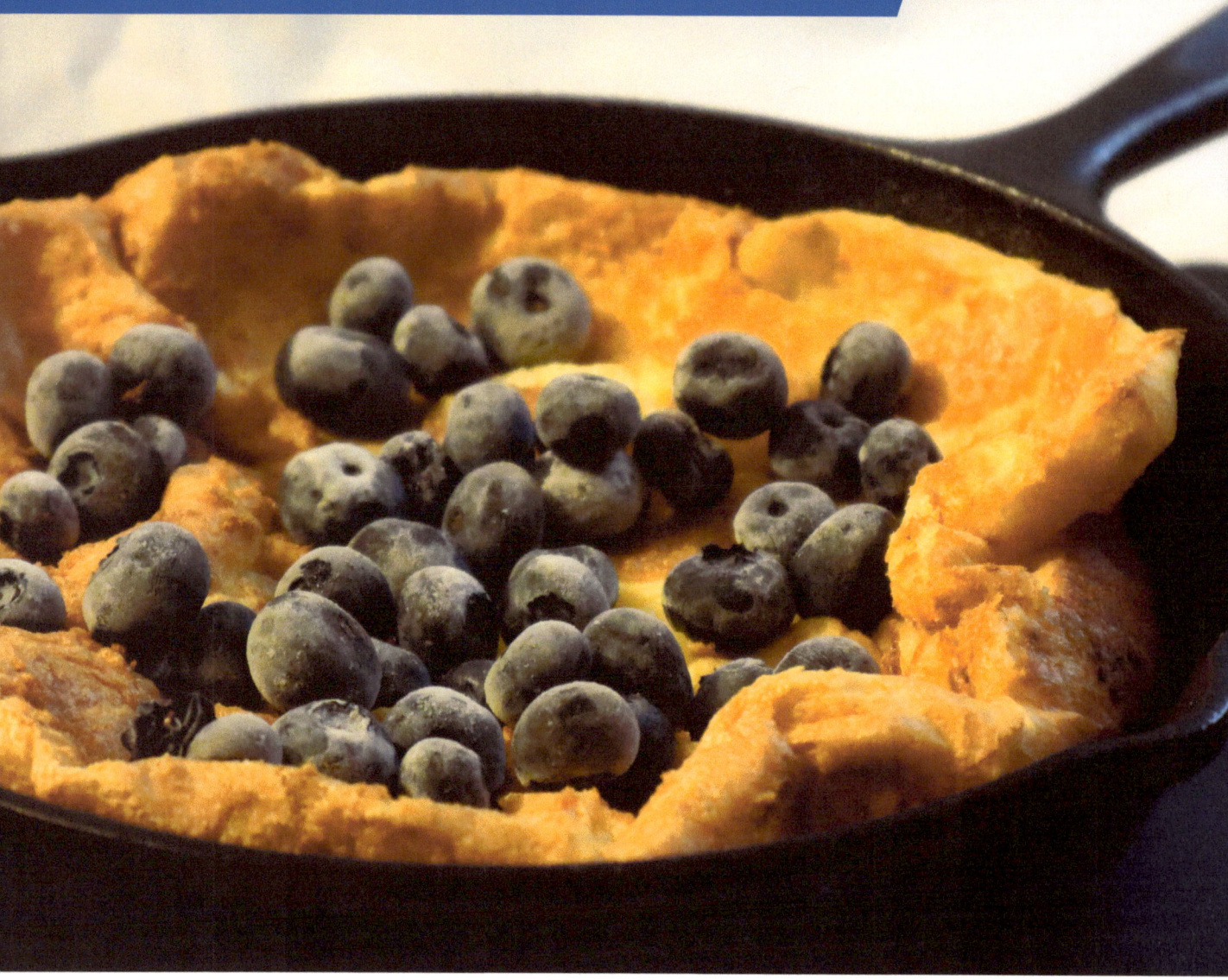

Is it a pancake? Is it a popover? This puffy, eggy concoction isn't always easy to describe but checks the boxes for delicious, scrumptious, and tasty. Enjoy plain for a simple delight, go for sweetness with berries, chocolate, or powdered sugar, or opt for savory with cheese, meat, or herb additions. It's hard to go wrong, whatever you choose.

Serving:
2 people

Prep Time:
5 minutes

Bake Time:
20 minutes

Breakfast

Ingredients

- 4 eggs
- 1 cup milk
- 1 cup flour
- ¼ tsp salt
- 1 tsp vanilla
- 3 tbsp butter

Directions

1. Preheat the oven to 425°F.
2. In a blender, mix eggs, milk, flour, salt, and vanilla until smooth.
3. Place butter in a 12-inch cast iron pan or 9x9 pan and set in the oven until melted.
4. Pour batter into the pan with melted butter and bake for 20 minutes or until golden brown and puffy.
5. Top with syrup, powdered sugar, or toppings of choice.

Variations

- Make a sweet version by adding chopped fruit or chocolate chips to batter.
    - Apples and cinnamon
    - Blueberries
    - Raspberries and chocolate chips
    - Peach chunks
    - Chocolate chips and peanut butter chips
- Make a savory version by adding shredded cheese, herbs, meat, or veggies to batter.

Double Recipe (4 people)

- 8 eggs
- 2 cups milk
- 2 cups flour
- ½ tsp salt
- 2 tsp vanilla
- 6 tbsp butter

(Use two cast iron pans or two 9x9 pans)

Single Serve (1 person)

- 2 eggs
- ½ cup milk
- ½ cup flour
- Pinch of salt
- ½ tsp vanilla
- 1 ½ tbsp butter

(Use 10-inch cast iron pan or similar smaller pan)

Apple Peanut Butter Scones with Apple Cinnamon Icing

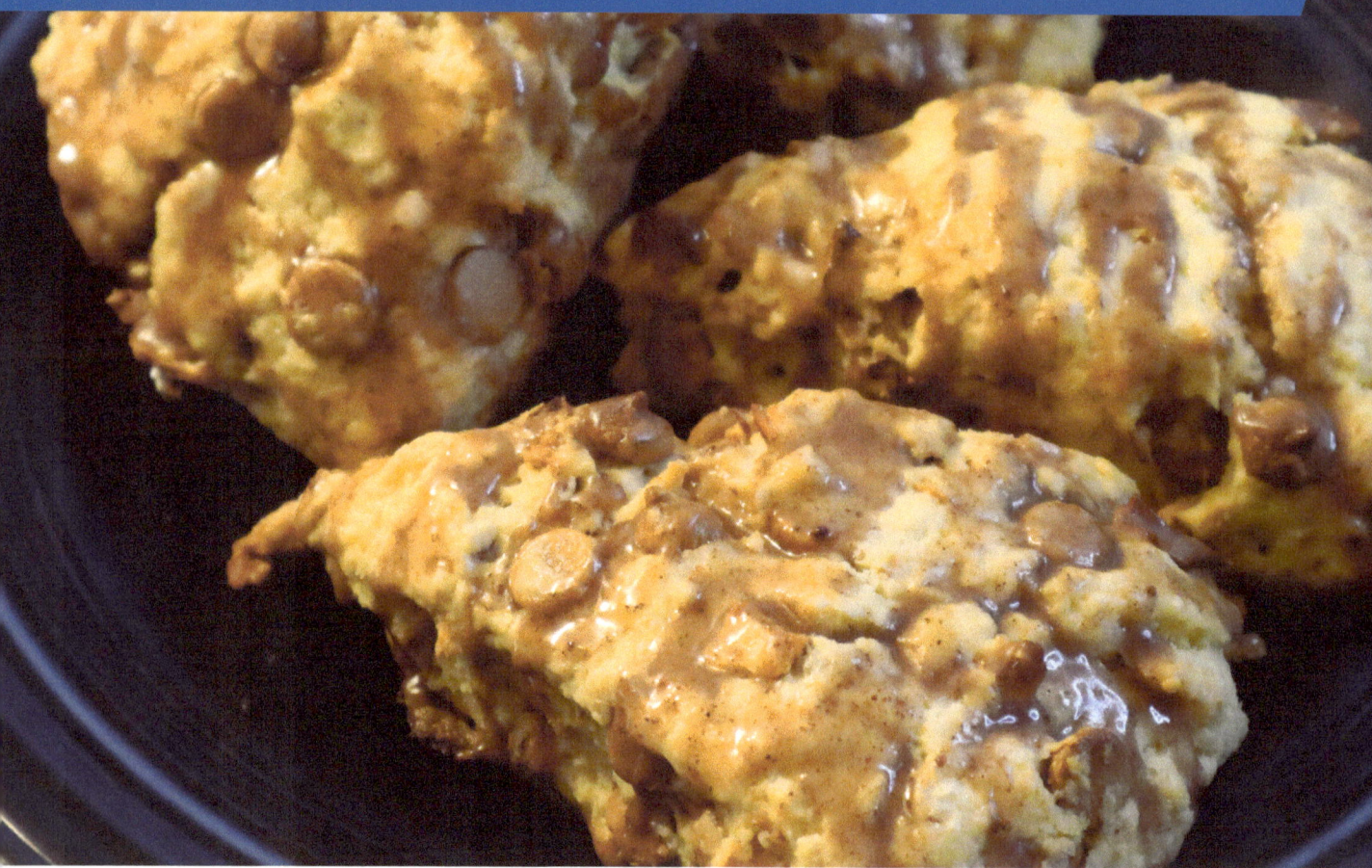

A tasty twist on the classic apples and peanut butter snack. Bits of sweet apple mixed with chips of peanut butter delivered in a warm, soft scone topped with cinnamon icing. Easy to make and hard to resist, enjoy for breakfast, an afternoon snack, dessert, or a bite before bedtime. I'll bet it's better than that flat, flavor-lacking scone from Starbucks.

Serving:
8 scones

Prep Time:
10 minutes

Bake Time:
20 minutes

Ingredients

- 2 ½ cups flour
- ½ tsp salt
- ¼ cup granulated sugar
- 2 ¼ tsp baking powder
- 6 tbsp cold unsalted butter, cubed
- ¾ cup heavy whipping cream, plus extra for topping
- 2 large eggs
- 2 tsp vanilla
- 1 cup diced apples
- ¾ cup PB baking chips
- 1 tsp cinnamon
- 2 cups powdered sugar
- ⅛ – ¼ cup warmed apple cider (or apple juice)
- Dash of nutmeg

Note:

Water can be substituted for apple cider/juice.

Can use dried apples in place of diced apples.

Directions

1. Preheat the oven to 400°F. Line baking sheet with parchment paper.
2. Whisk together flour, salt, granulated sugar, and baking powder.
3. Add in cubed butter and work into flour with fingers until all or most lumps are gone and mixture resembles damp sand.
4. In a separate bowl, whisk together heavy whipping cream, eggs, and vanilla.
5. Add wet ingredients to dry and stir several times.
6. Add in apples and PB chips and gently mix until a loose but moist dough forms (the less you stir, the lighter the scone).
7. Transfer dough to a well-floured surface and gather into a roughly 8-in circle, about ¾ of an inch thick.
8. Cut into 8 wedges.
9. Place wedges on lined baking sheet with 1-2 inches of space between.
10. Brush top of scones with heavy whipping cream.
11. Bake for about 20 minutes until golden brown.

Glaze

12. While scones are baking, warm apple cider (or juice).
13. Mix powdered sugar, cinnamon and nutmeg.
14. Slowly add apple cider to the sugar mixture until it reaches the consistency you desire.
15. Once scones are baked, drizzle glaze over scones and enjoy!

Apple Peanut Butter Scones
continued

Variations

- 2 tsp of cinnamon (instead of apples/PB)
- Chocolate chips
- Blueberries/raspberries/etc.
- Chunks of various fruits
- Almonds/pecans/walnuts/pumpkin seeds
- Lemon zest + blueberries or raspberries

Glaze Variations:

- Use water and plain powdered sugar.
- Drizzle with melted chocolate or PB.
- Sprinkle with coarse sugar.
- Use lemon juice/zest and powdered sugar.

Double Recipe (16 scones)

- 5 cups flour
- 1 tsp salt
- ½ cup granulated sugar
- 4 ½ tsp baking powder
- 12 tbsp cold unsalted butter, cubed
- 1 ½ cups heavy whipping cream, plus extra for topping
- 4 large eggs
- 4 tsp vanilla
- 2 cups diced apples
- 1 ½ cups PB baking chips
- 2 tsp cinnamon
- 4 cups powdered sugar
- ¼ – ½ cup warmed apple cider (or apple juice)
- ¼ tsp of nutmeg

Single Serve (4 scones)

- 1 ¼ cups flour
- ¼ tsp salt
- ⅛ cup granulated sugar
- 1 ⅛ tsp baking powder
- 3 tbsp cold unsalted butter, cubed
- ½ cup and 2 tbsp heavy whipping cream, plus extra for topping
- 1 large egg
- 1 tsp vanilla
- ½ cup diced apples
- ½ cup and 2 tbsp PB baking chips
- ½ tsp cinnamon
- 1 cup powdered sugar
- ⅛ cup warmed apple cider (or apple juice)
- Dash of nutmeg

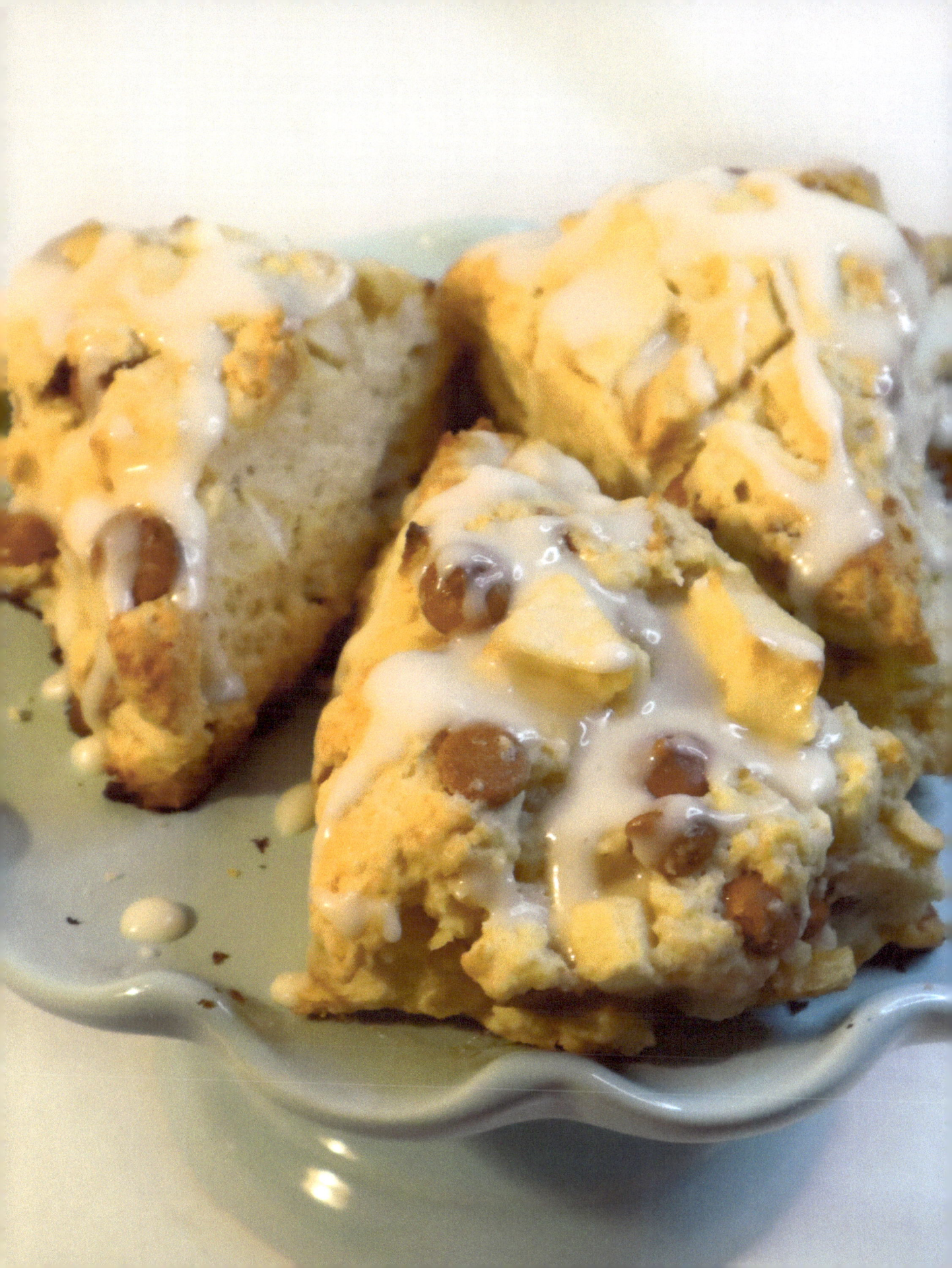

Blueberry Muffins

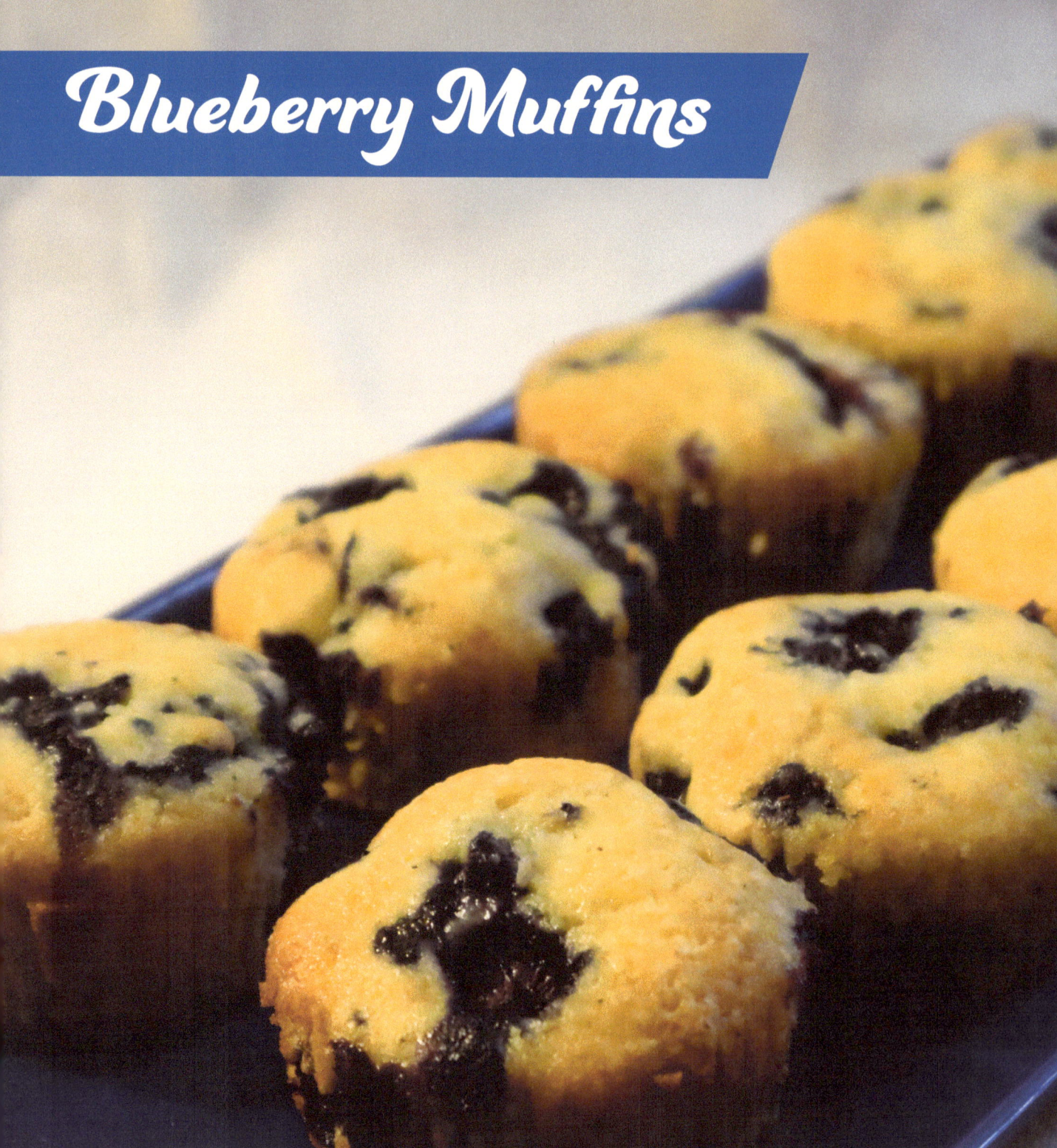

Packed with juicy, sweet blueberries for a quick and easy on-the-go snack. Or a slow, savoring breakfast with your morning coffee or tea to start the day. However, you enjoy it, it's a classic for a reason. Mmmmm.

Serving:
5 jumbo, 10 regular

Prep Time:
10 minutes

Bake Time:
30 minutes

Breakfast

Ingredients

- 1 cup flour
- 1 tsp baking powder
- ¼ tsp salt
- ¼ cup softened butter
- ½ cup + 1 tbsp sugar, divided
- 1 large egg
- ¼ cup milk
- ½ tsp vanilla
- 1 ½ cups blueberries

Directions

1. Preheat oven to 375°F and line muffin pan with paper liners.
2. Combine flour, baking powder, and salt in bowl
3. Beat butter and ½ cup sugar in a large mixing bowl until light and fluffy.
4. Add egg and beat well.
5. Add dry ingredients, alternating with milk and vanilla—begin and end with dry.
6. Toss blueberries in 1 tbsp sugar and fold into batter. (Batter will be thick.)
7. Fill muffin cups about ⅔ full and bake for 25-30 minutes until lightly browned on top and toothpick comes out clean.

Variations

- Substitute blueberries with berries or fruit chunks of choice.
- Substitute chocolate chips and/or peanut butter chips.
- Leave out blueberries and add 1-2 teaspoons of cinnamon.

Double Recipe
(9 jumbo, 18 regular)

- 2 cups flour
- 2 tsp baking powder
- ½ tsp salt
- ½ cup softened butter
- 1 cup + 2 tbsp sugar, divided
- 2 large eggs
- ½ cup milk
- 1 tsp vanilla
- 2 ½ cups blueberries

Single Serve
(3 jumbo, 5 regular)

- ½ cup flour
- ½ tsp baking powder
- ⅛ tsp salt
- 2 tbsp softened butter
- ¼ cup + 1 tsp sugar, divided
- ½ large egg
- 2 tbsp milk
- ¼ tsp vanilla
- ¾ cup blueberries

Crusty Artisan Bread

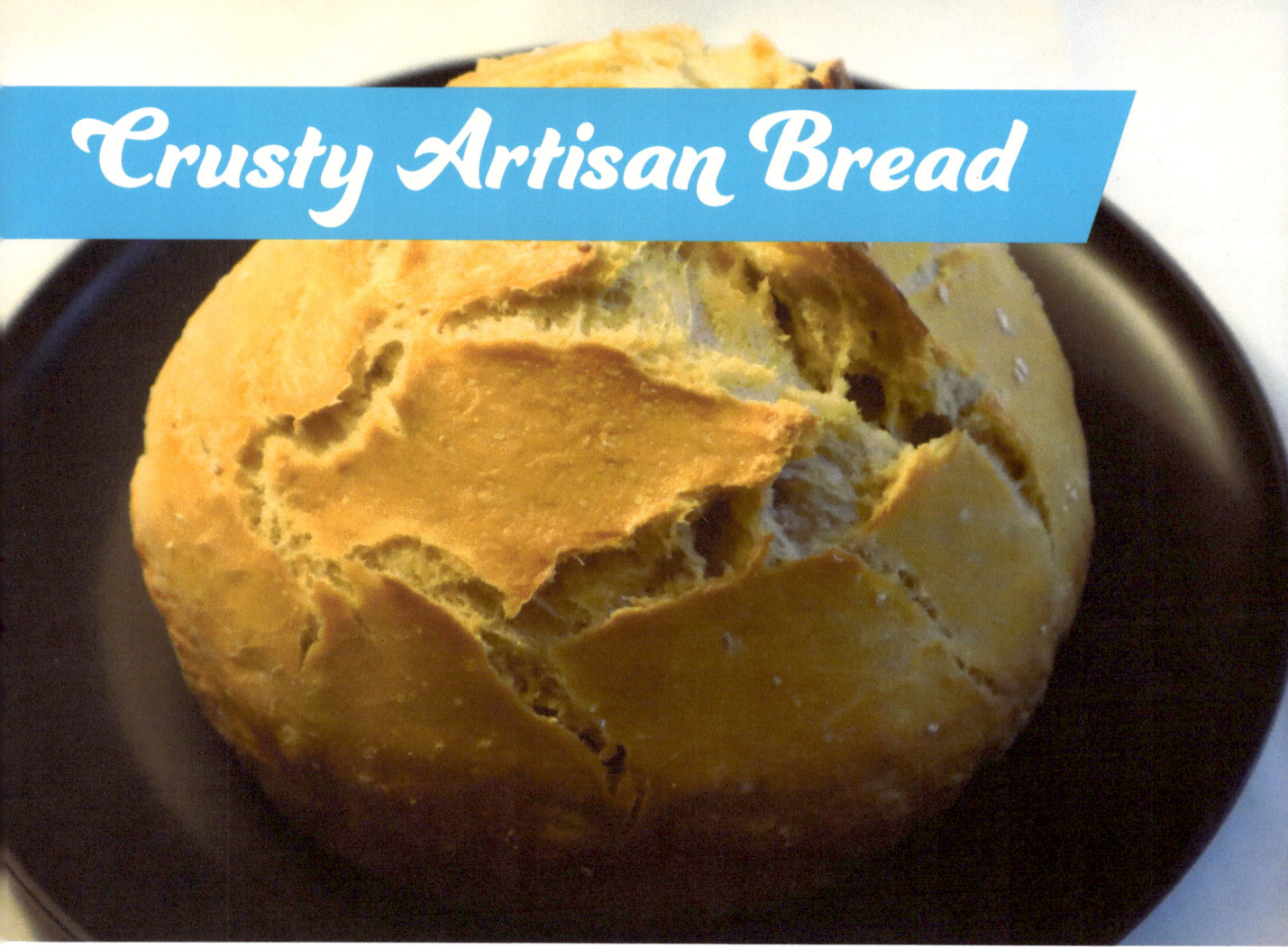

Crusty on the outside, soft and tender on the inside—this loaf is tasty when enjoyed warm with melty butter or stuffed with your favorite sandwich fixings. However you eat it, it's hard to go wrong. Plus, your home will smell like a bakery. What's not to love?

Serving:
1 loaf

Prep Time:
5 minutes

Bake Time:
45 minutes

Ingredients

- 3 cups flour
- 1 tsp dry active yeast
- 1 ½ tsp salt
- 1 ½ cups lukewarm water

Directions

1. In a large bowl, stir together the flour, salt and yeast. Stir in water using a wooden spoon until the mixture forms a shaggy but cohesive dough. Do not overwork the dough. The less you "work" it, the more soft, fluffy air pockets will form. Stir in desired mix-in ingredients now.*
2. Cover bowl tightly with plastic wrap. Let dough sit at room temperature for 8-24 hours.** Dough will bubble up and rise.
3. After the dough is ready, preheat the oven to 450°F. Place your Dutch oven (or other large baking dish), uncovered, into the preheated oven for 30 minutes.
4. While your Dutch oven preheats, turn dough onto a well-floured surface. With floured hands, form the dough into a ball. Cover dough loosely with plastic wrap and let rest.
5. After the 30 minutes are up, carefully remove Dutch oven. With floured hands, place dough into it. (You can put a piece of parchment under the dough if your Dutch oven isn't enamel coated.)
6. Replace cover and bake for 30 minutes. Then, carefully remove cover and bake for 7-15 minutes*** more, uncovered.
7. Carefully remove loaf to a cooling rack.
8. Enjoy!

Variations

Mix-Ins:

- Cranberries and pumpkin seeds
- Garlic and herbs
- Dried fruit
- Nuts and seeds
- Cheese (cheddar, asiago, etc.)

I recommend adding these mix-ins to the dough when you first mix it up.

> **Note:**
> ***Uncovered baking time depends on your oven. Just keep an eye on it!
>
> Heating your Dutch oven to 450°F will not damage it, or the knob on top.
>
> **Dough can rise anywhere between 8-24 hours and it will bake up beautifully.
>
> You can use any large oven-safe dish and cover if you don't have Dutch oven.

Double Recipe (2 loaves)

- 6 cups flour
- 2 tsp dry active yeast
- 3 tsp salt
- 3 cups lukewarm water

Single Serve (half loaf)

- 1 ½ cups flour
- ½ tsp dry active yeast
- ¾ tsp salt
- ¾ cups lukewarm water

Buttery Garlic Breadsticks

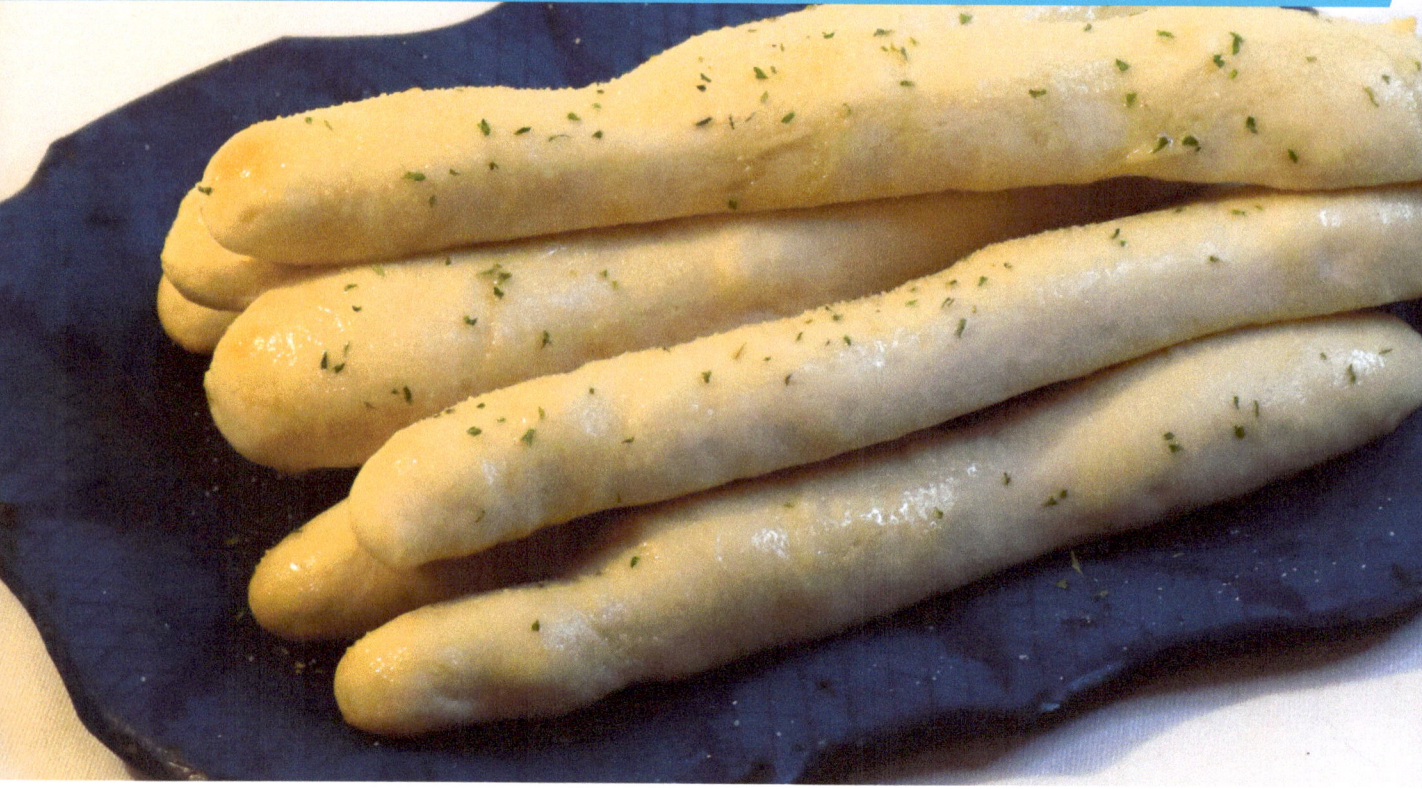

Soft, buttery, garlicky breadsticks. A yummy compliment to soup or pasta. Breadsticks are one of my favorites and these are light and damn near melt-in-your mouth delicious. Add garlic until you feel that in your soul. (Is there ever too much garlic?)

Serving:
16 breadsticks

Prep Time:
2 hours, 15 minutes

Bake Time:
10 minutes

Ingredients

- 1 cup warm water
- 2 tbsp sugar
- 2 tsp dry active yeast
- 2 ½ – 3 cups bread flour
- 1 ½ tsp salt
- ¼ cup softened butter (4 tbsp)
- 3 tbsp melted butter
- 1 tsp garlic salt
- 1 tsp dried parsley

Directions

1. In a small bowl, mix sugar in warm water until dissolved and add yeast. Let sit until foamy, about 5 minutes.
2. Whisk together 2 ½ cups bread flour and salt.
3. Add softened butter to flour in chunks and blend until well combined.
4. Add yeast mixture and knead with dough hook for about 5-8 minutes. If sticky, add additional flour a tablespoon at a time until stops sticking to the sides.
5. Place dough in a lightly greased bowl and cover. Let rise for about 1 hour or until doubled in size.
6. Once dough has risen, remove and roll into a long log. Divide into approximately 16 equal pieces.
7. Roll each piece to approximately 6-7 inches long.
8. Place dough sticks onto parchment lined baking sheets, cover with a clean tea towel, and let rise again for an hour or until doubled in size.
9. Preheat the oven to 400°F.
10. Bake breadsticks for about 10 minutes, or until beginning to lightly brown.
11. Combine melted butter, garlic salt, and parsley. Just after breadsticks come out of the oven, brush on herbed butter generously with a pastry brush.
12. Enjoy!

Variations

- Sprinkle with cinnamon sugar for a sweet alternative.
- Shape into rolls instead of breadsticks.

Note: Breadsticks can be frozen (skip adding garlic butter). Let thaw, then heat up and add garlic butter.

Double Recipe (32 breadsticks)

- 2 cups warm water
- ¼ cup sugar
- 4 tsp dry active yeast
- 5 – 5 ½ cups bread flour
- 3 tsp salt
- ½ cup softened butter (8 tbsp)
- 6 tbsp melted butter
- 2 tsp garlic salt
- 2 tsp dried parsley

Single Serve (8 breadsticks)

- ½ cup warm water
- 1 tbsp sugar
- 1 tsp dry active yeast
- 1 ¼ – 1 ½ cups bread flour
- ¾ tsp salt
- 2 tbsp softened butter
- 2 tbsp melted butter
- ½ tsp garlic salt
- ½ tsp dried parsley

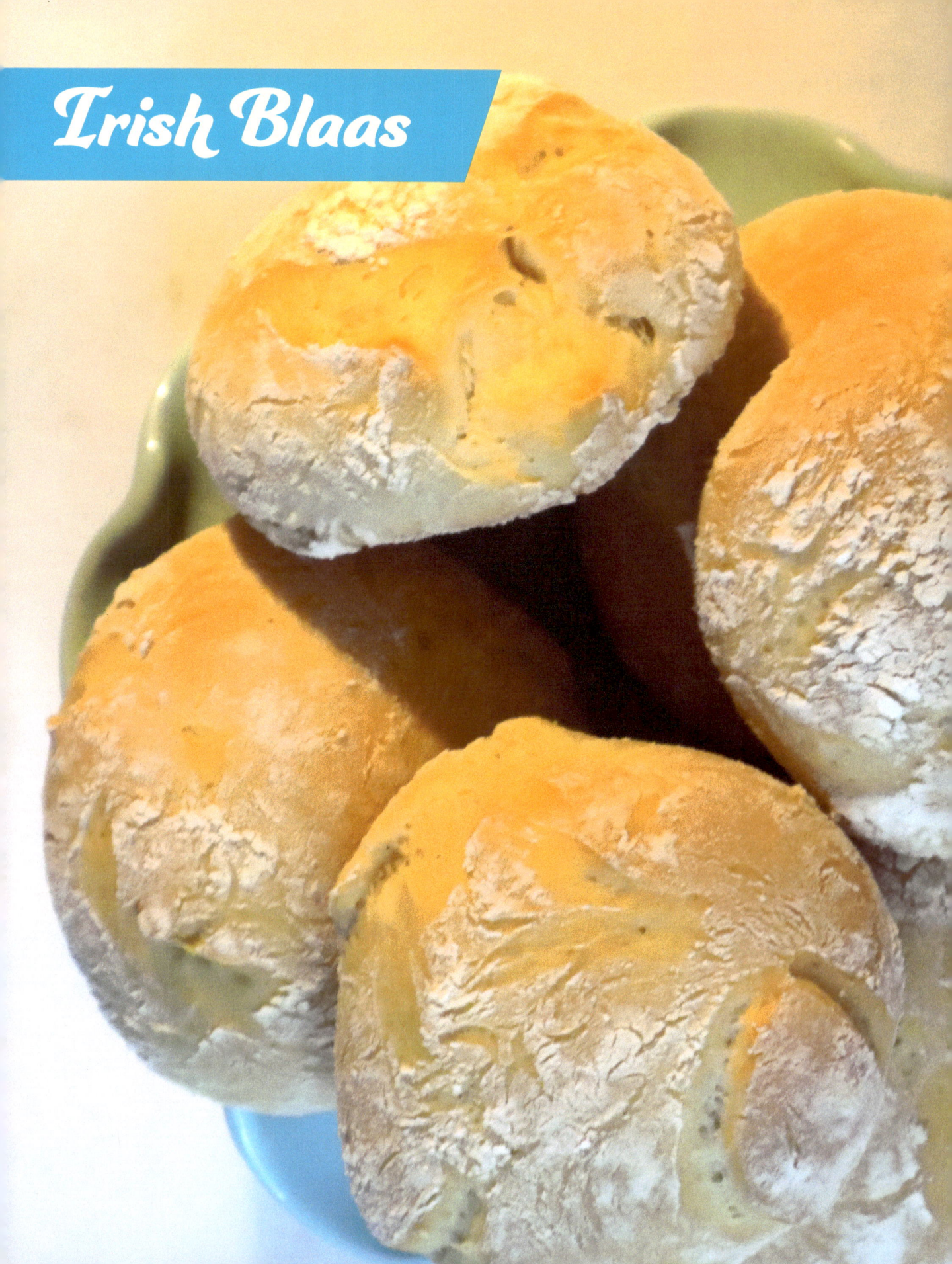

My friend Rachel says that the true test of good bread is eating it without toppings or condiments. She's absolutely right. These soft, pillowy rolls are simple yet incredibly tasty—even before you add butter or sandwich fillings. Despite their name, these are anything but blah!

Serving:
12 rolls

Prep Time:
20 minutes

Bake Time:
18 minutes

Ingredients

- 2 ¼ tsp dry active yeast
- 1 tbsp sugar
- ½ tsp salt
- ½ cup softened butter (1 stick)
- 1 ½ cups warm water
- 4 cups flour + ½ cup flour

Directions

1. Mix yeast, sugar, and warm water to the mixer bowl. Let sit for about 5 minutes until foamy.
2. Add 4 cups flour, salt, and butter (in chunks). Knead for about 5 minutes, until the dough gets a bit of a shine, will be sticky) and pulls away from the sides of the bowl.
3. Cover dough and let rise for 1 hour or until doubled in size.
4. Roll dough into a large log. Divide into 12 equal pieces.
5. Shape each piece into a round and roll through ½ cup of flour. Set on a parchment lined baking sheet.
6. Cover and let rise again until doubled.
7. Preheat the oven to 400°F.
8. Bake for 18-22 minutes until lightly browned and they sound slightly hollow when tapped.

Double Recipe (24 rolls)

- 4 ½ tsp dry active yeast
- 2 tbsp sugar
- 1 tsp salt
- 1 cup softened butter (2 sticks)
- 3 cups warm water
- 8 cups flour + 1 cup flour

Single Serve (6 rolls)

- 1 rounded tsp dry active yeast
- ⅓ tbsp sugar
- ¼ tsp salt
- ¼ cup softened butter (½ stick)
- ¾ cup warm water
- 2 cups flour + ¼ cup flour

Banana Bread

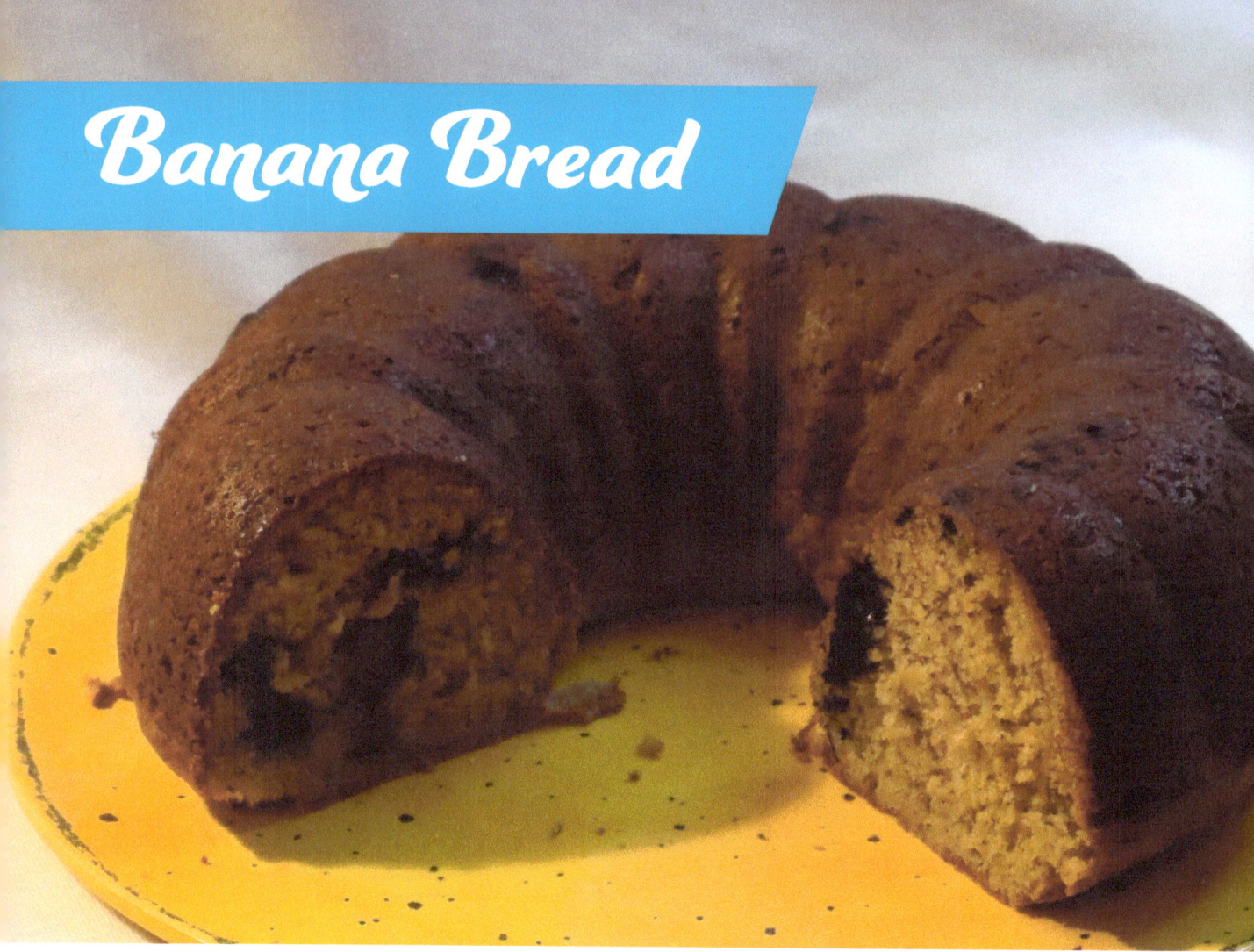

Another classic. The savior of brown bananas everywhere. Delicious in loaf form, muffin form, or bundt form. My secret trick to top notch banana bread? Stick it in the freezer overnight (or longer) before slicing in. The flavors really explode and the moisture is perfect after a bit of freezing!

Serving:
1 loaf

Prep Time:
10 minutes

Bake Time:
1 hour

Ingredients

- ½ cup softened butter (1 stick)
- 1 cup sugar
- 2 eggs
- 1 cup banana
- 1 ¾ cups flour
- 1 tsp vanilla
- 1 tsp lemon juice
- ½ package cream cheese (4 oz)
- ½ tsp salt
- 1 tsp baking soda
- 1 tsp baking powder

Directions

1. Preheat the oven to 350°F. Lightly grease loaf pan.
2. Cream butter and sugar until light and fluffy.
3. Blend in vanilla and lemon juice.
4. Add eggs, one at a time, mixing after each.
5. Mix remaining ingredients until combined.
6. Pour batter into loaf pan (about ¾ full).
7. Bake for about 1 hour until the toothpick inserted in the center comes out clean. (Baking times may vary by oven so adjust as needed.)

Variations

- Optional additions:
    - Nuts
    - Fruit
    - Chocolate chips
    - Peanut butter chips
    - For an extra delicious treat, chop up Reese's Cups and mix into batter.

> **Note:**
> Can bake in muffin tin, just reduce baking time as needed.

Double Recipe (2 loaves)

- 1 cup softened butter (2 sticks)
- 2 cups sugar
- 4 eggs
- 2 cups banana
- 3 ½ cups flour
- 2 tsp vanilla
- 2 tsp lemon juice
- 1 package cream cheese (8 oz)
- 1 tsp salt
- 2 tsp baking soda
- 2 tsp baking powder

Single Serve (mini loaf)

- ¼ cup softened butter (4 tbsp)
- ½ cup sugar
- 1 egg
- ½ cup banana
- ¾ cup and 2 tbsp flour
- ½ tsp vanilla
- ½ tsp lemon juice
- ¼ package cream cheese (2 oz)
- ¼ tsp salt
- ½ tsp baking soda
- ½ tsp baking powder

(Use mini loaf pan or muffin tins)

Garlic Pesto Pull-Apart Bread

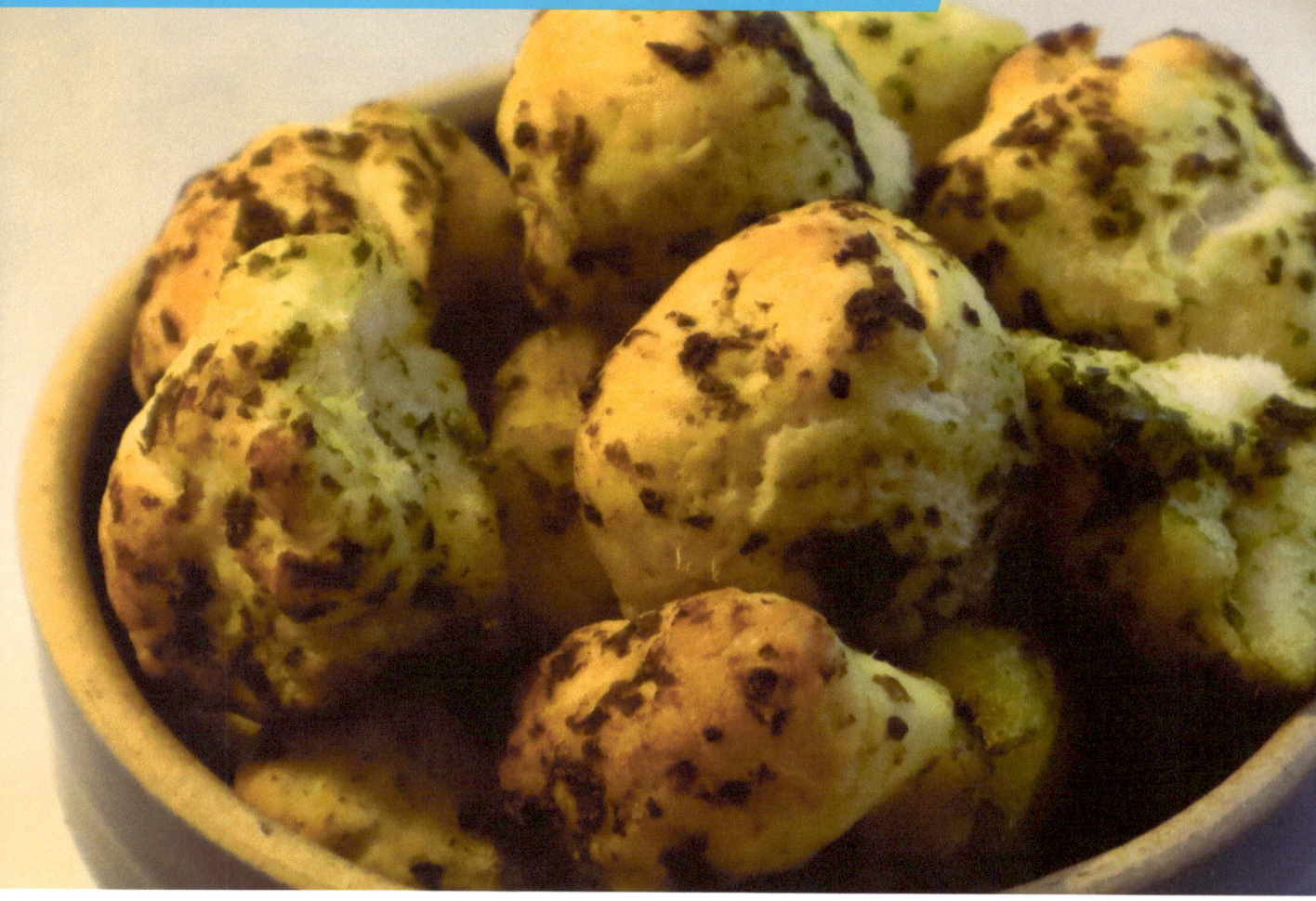

This recipe was born out of one of my mom's garlic & herb pull apart bread—with, in my opinion, a few upgrades (sorry, Mom!) Soft, buttery bread and garlicky pesto together in delicious bite-sized chunks baked to perfection. Pair it with your favorite pasta for sheer bliss in your mouth.

Serving:
2 people

Prep Time:
1 hour, 10 minutes

Bake Time:
10 minutes

Ingredients

- ½ cup warm water
- 1 tbsp sugar
- 1 tsp dry active yeast
- 1 ¼ – 1 ½ cups bread flour
- ¾ tsp salt
- 2 tbsp softened butter
- 2 tbsp pesto
- ½ tsp garlic salt

Directions

1. In a small bowl, mix sugar in warm water until dissolved and add yeast. Let sit until foamy, about 5 minutes.
2. Whisk together flour and salt.
3. Add softened butter to flour in chunks and blend until well combined.
4. Add yeast mixture and knead with dough hook for about 5-8 minutes. If sticky, add additional flour a tablespoon at a time until stops sticking to the sides.
5. Divide dough into ½ to 1 inch pieces.
6. Mix garlic salt with pesto.
7. Dunk dough pieces in pesto and drop into bundt pan (if no bundt pan, use aluminum foil or an oven safe dish to create hole in center).
8. Cover with a tea towel and let rise for about 1 hour or until doubled in size.
9. Preheat the oven to 400°F.
10. Bake for about 10-15 minutes, or until lightly browned and baked through.
11. Let cool slightly and enjoy by pulling off bite sized dough chunks!

Variations

- Can substitute melted butter and herbs for pesto.
- Add Parmesan cheese for cheesy version.

Double Recipe (4 people)

- 1 cup warm water
- 2 tbsp sugar
- 2 tsp dry active yeast
- 3 cups bread flour
- 1 ½ tsp salt
- 4 tbsp softened butter
- 4 tbsp pesto
- 1 tsp garlic salt

Single Serve (1 person)

- ¼ cup warm water
- ½ tbsp sugar
- ½ tsp dry active yeast
- ¾ – 1 cup bread flour
- ⅓ tsp salt
- 1 tbsp softened butter
- 1 tbsp pesto
- ¼ tsp garlic salt

Garlic Herb Flatbread (Naan)

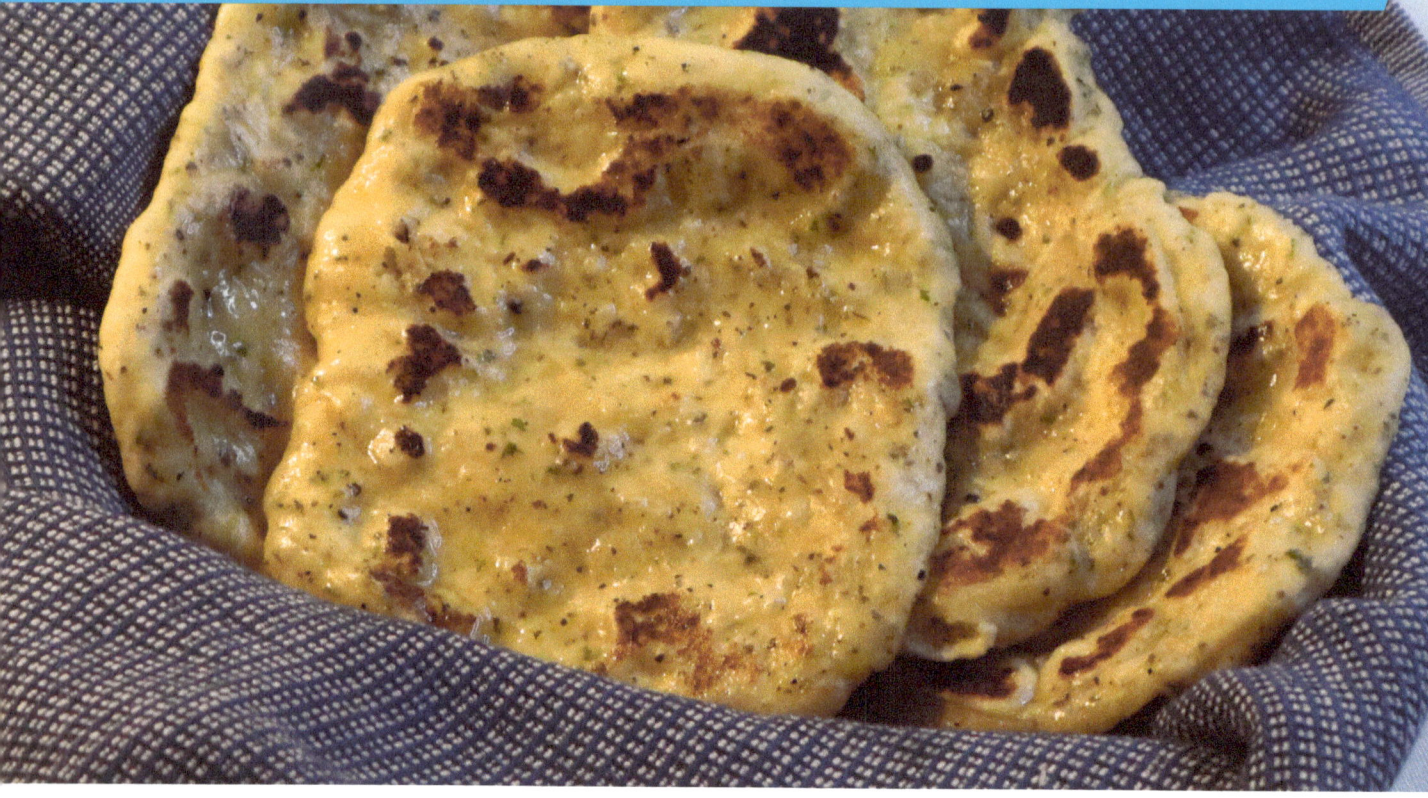

It's **homemade** Naan. And it's surprisingly easy to make. What else need I say? Except perhaps to recommend using it to make grilled cheese sandwiches (seriously, you won't regret it).

Serving:
8 flatbreads

Prep Time:
1 hour, 30 minutes

Bake Time:
15 minutes

Ingredients

- 1 ½ cups flour
- ¾ cup bread flour
- ½ cup + 2 tbsp warm water
- 5 tbsp plain Greek yogurt
- 2 tbsp + 2 tbsp melted butter, divided in half
- 1 ½ tsp instant yeast
- 1 tsp sugar
- 1 tsp salt
- 1 rounded tsp parsley
- 1 rounded tsp oregano
- 1 ½ tsp garlic salt
- Other herbs as desired

Directions

1. Combine all ingredients and mix until shaggy.
2. Knead dough until smooth, bouncy, and slightly tacky.
3. Place in a greased bowl, cover, and let rise for about an hour, or until doubled in size.
4. Divide dough into 8 equal pieces. Shape each into a ball, cover, and let rest for 20-30 minutes.
5. Preheat a cast iron pan or electric griddle over medium-high heat until very hot.
6. On a lightly floured or greased surface, roll each ball into either a 6-7 inch or 8-9 inch round, depending on desired thickness. Keep other pieces covered while working.
7. Cook naan for 30-40 seconds, covered, until bubbles form on top and underside browns. Flip over to brown the other side for 30-40 seconds.
8. Remove bread from pan, brush with melted butter. Keep wrapped in a towel in an airtight container until ready to serve.

Variations

- Can substitute various herbs as desired.
- For cheesy stuffed herbed naan, add shredded cheese to rounds, fold over, and roll out as instructed.
- Add herbs to melted butter for brushing for stronger flavors.

Note:

Will keep in an airtight container at room temp for several days. Can freeze for longer.

Vanilla flavored Greek yogurt can be used if you don't have plain on hand.

Double Recipe (16 flatbreads)

- 3 cups flour
- 1 ½ cups bread flour
- 1 ¼ cups warm water
- ½ cup + 2 tbsp plain Greek yogurt
- 4 tbsp + 4 tbsp melted butter, divided in half
- 3 tsp instant yeast
- 2 tsp sugar
- 2 tsp salt
- 2 rounded tsp parsley
- 2 rounded tsp oregano
- 3 tsp garlic salt
- Other herbs as desired

Single Serve (4 flatbreads)

- ¾ cups flour
- ¼ cup + 2 tbsp bread flour
- ¼ cup + 1 tbsp warm water
- 3 ½ tbsp plain Greek yogurt
- 1 tbsp + 1 tbsp melted butter, divided in half
- ¾ tsp instant yeast
- ½ tsp sugar
- ½ tsp salt
- ½ rounded tsp parsley
- ½ rounded tsp oregano
- ¾ tsp garlic salt
- Other herbs as desired

Pita Bread

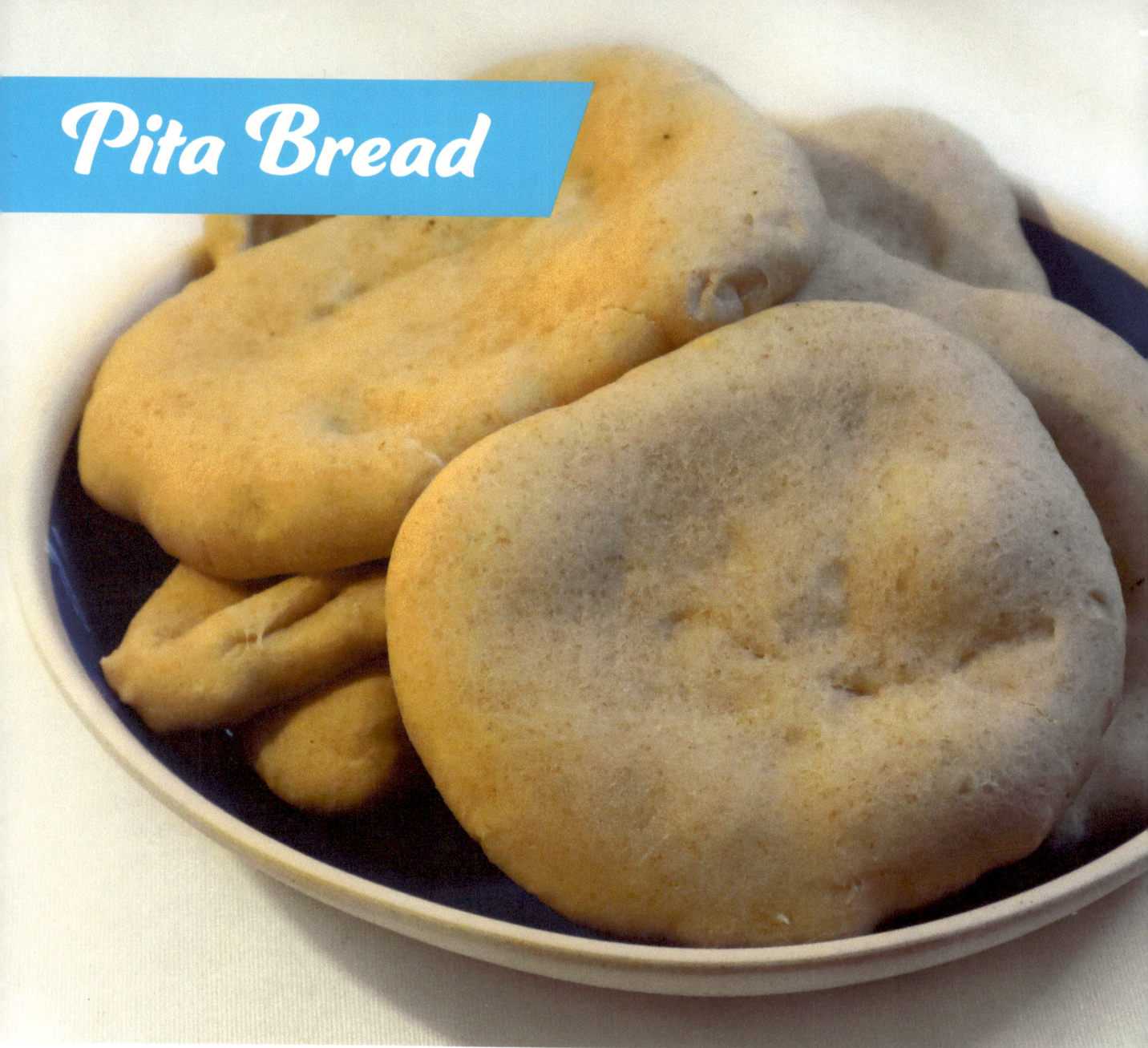

I'm not gonna lie, getting my pitas to puff properly took many (many) failed attempts. I still don't always get it right. But the pride when I see them balloon up? Immense and always comes with a happy kitchen dance. And, honestly, even if I "fail" and it doesn't puff, the bread tastes much like naan so really one can't lose. Enjoy your win, puff or no puff!

Serving:
10 pitas

Prep Time:
3 hour, 30 minutes

Bake Time:
3-5 minutes

Ingredients

- 2 cups flour
- ½ cup whole wheat flour
- 1 tbsp sugar
- 1 tsp salt
- 1 tbsp olive oil
- 2 tsp instant yeast
- 1 cup warm water

Note:

Best warm and fresh, but will keep in an airtight container for several days or be frozen for several weeks.

Whole wheat flour is optional, can just be replaced with regular flour.

Directions

1. Combine both flours, salt, and sugar in a mixing bowl.
2. Add yeast to warm water and stir to dissolve completely.
3. Pour into a mixing bowl, add olive oil and combine all into a sticky mess.
4. Knead for 8-10 minutes until soft and tacky.
5. Lightly oil bowl and cover. Let proof for about 2 hours.
6. After 2 hours, gently deflate and divide into 10 equal pieces. Form into slightly flat rounds and cover with a damp tea towel.
7. Take the first round and roll thinly and evenly to about 6 inches. Place on a parchment paper lined baking sheet and cover with another damp tea towel.
8. Once all are rolled out and covered, let rest for an additional 30 minutes.
9. Preheat the oven to 345°F with a baking stone or upside down baking sheet inside.
10. Once hot, flip rolled out dough (opposite side up) onto the hot pan and bake for 3-5 minutes until nicely puffed up.
11. Wrap in a tea towel directly from the oven to keep it soft.
12. Eat and enjoy!

Double Recipe (20 pitas)

- 4 cups flour
- 1 cup whole wheat flour
- 2 tbsp sugar
- 2 tsp salt
- 2 tbsp olive oil
- 4 tsp instant yeast
- 2 cups warm water

Single Serve (5 pitas)

- 1 cup flour
- ¼ cup whole wheat flour
- ½ tbsp sugar
- ½ tsp salt
- ½ tbsp olive oil
- 1 tsp instant yeast
- ½ cup warm water

Soft Pretzels

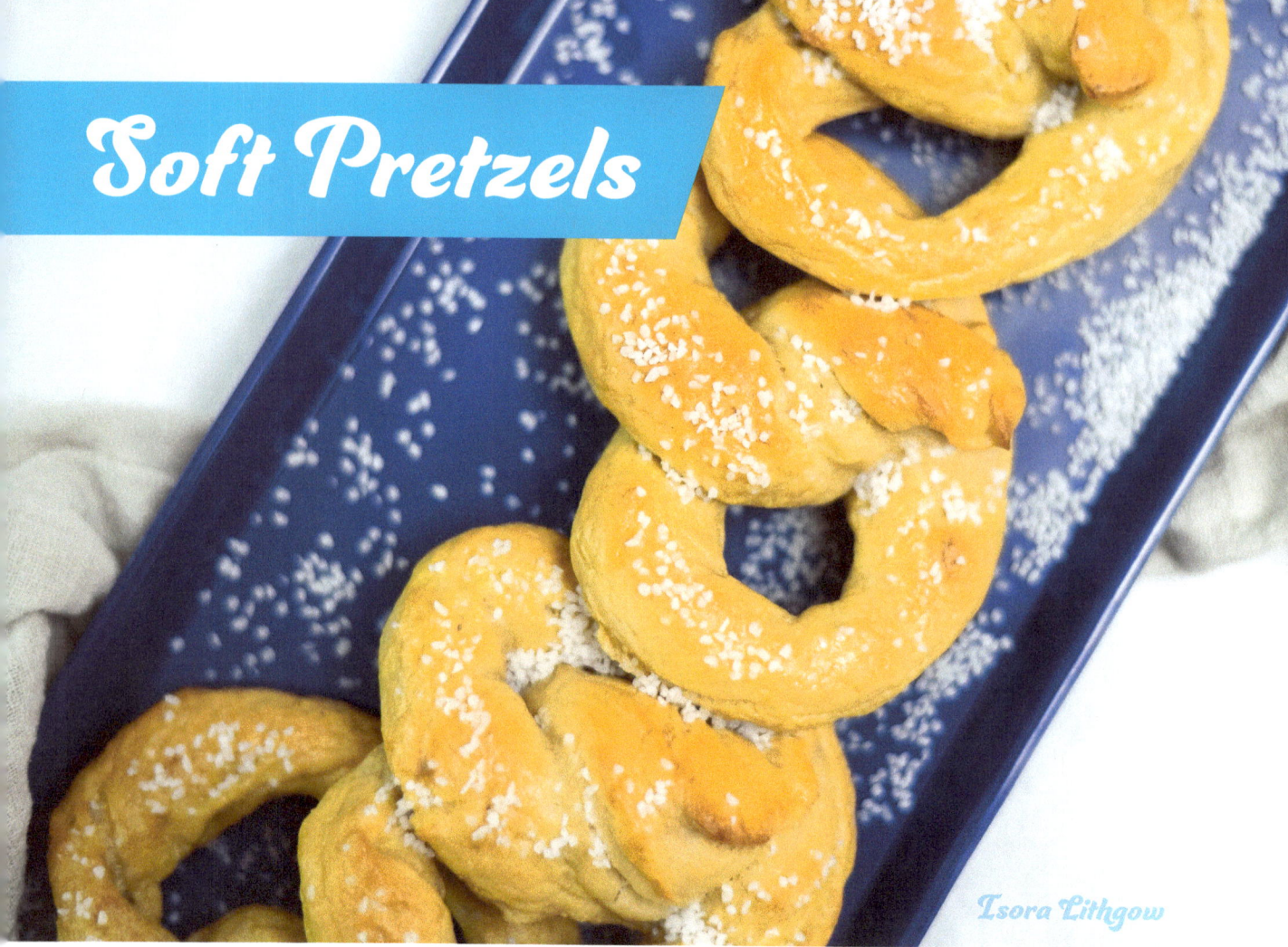

Isora Lithgow

Soft pretzels bring up a rather random assortment of memories for me—going to the fair, Auntie Anne's in the mall, baseball games, my favorite pizza place (Mellow Mushroom) in Asheville, NC, and my friend, Eireann. This recipe is the closest I've come to recreating my favorite pretzel bites from Mellow Mushroom. Chewy, full of flavor, and salty goodness in every bite. Yum!

Serving:
6 large pretzels

Prep Time:
50 minutes

Bake Time:
10 minutes

Ingredients

- ¾ cup warm water
- ½ tbsp molasses
- 2 ¼ tsp dry active yeast
- 1 ¾ cups flour
- 1 tsp salt
- ½ tbsp olive oil
- ¼ cup baking soda
- Egg wash
- Pretzel salt

Directions

1. Mix warm water and molasses until dissolved. Add yeast and let sit until foamy (about 5 minutes).
2. Add flour and salt to the mixer/bowl and whisk together.
3. Add wet ingredients and olive oil to the flour mixture.
4. Knead on low with a dough hook for about 5 minutes until tacky and smooth.
5. Form into a ball and place in a lightly greased bowl.
6. Cover and let rise for about 30 minutes (until doubled in size).
7. Preheat the oven to 525°F.
8. Shape dough into a log and cut into 6 equal pieces.
9. Roll each piece into a long strip and twist into pretzel shape.
10. Boil a large pot of water and slowly add ¼ cup baking soda (it will foam and bubble!)
11. Boil pretzels for 30 seconds to 1 minute.
12. Brush with egg wash and sprinkle with pretzel salt.
13. Bake for 8-9 minutes until browned.
14. ENJOY!

Variations

- Instead of pretzel salt, you can also brush with butter and toss with garlic salt and grated Parmesan cheese or cinnamon sugar after baking!
- Instead of shaping into a traditional pretzel shape, it can also be cut into small pretzel nuggets.

Note:
Dough can be frozen after rising. Just thaw, shape, boil, and bake.

Double Recipe (12 pretzels)

- 1 ½ cups warm water
- 1-2 tbsp molasses
- 4 ½ tsp dry active yeast
- 3 ½ cups flour
- 2 tsp salt
- 1 tbsp olive oil
- ¼ cup baking soda
- Egg wash
- Pretzel salt

Single Serve (3 pretzels)

- ½ cup and 2 tbsp warm water
- 1 tsp molasses
- 1 ⅛ tsp dry active yeast
- ¾ cup and 2 tbsp flour
- ½ tsp salt
- 1 ½ tsp olive oil
- ¼ cup baking soda
- Egg wash
- Pretzel salt

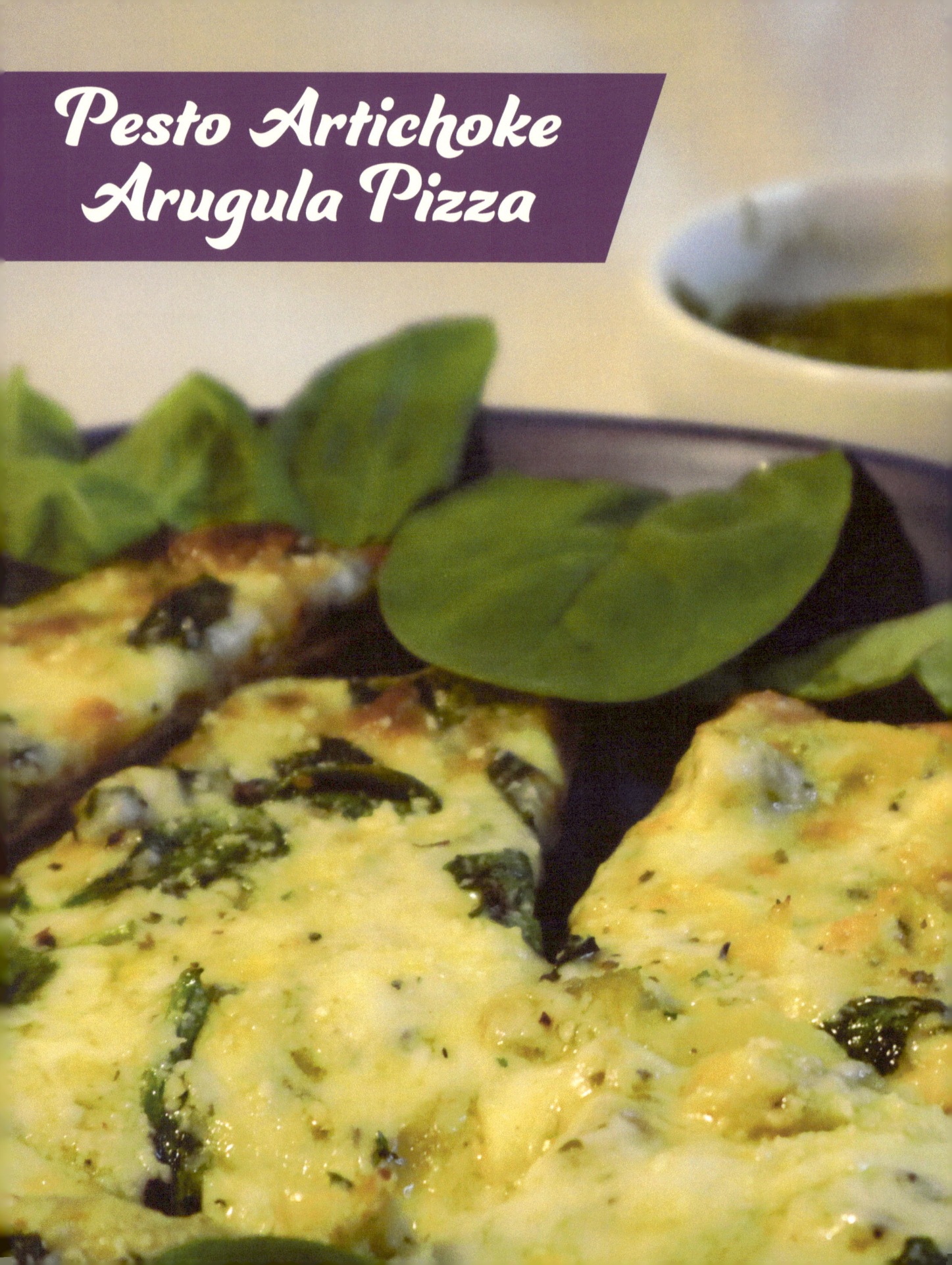

*I love pizza. I mean, I **really** love pizza. I could eat it every day and be perfectly happy. This recipe is my favorite—crispy, flavorful crust, garlicky pesto & herbs, peppery arugula, tasty artichokes, and oodles of cheese. Topped with Parmesan. Lots of Parmesan. There is no such thing as too much Parm.*

Serving:
1 large crust or 2 small crusts

Prep Time:
1 hour, 20 minutes

Bake Time:
10 minutes

Ingredients

Crust
- ¾ cup warm water
- ½ tbsp molasses
- 2 ¼ tsp dry active yeast
- 1 ¾ cups flour
- 1 tsp salt
- ½ tbsp olive oil
- 1 tbsp grated Parmesan cheese (optional)

Toppings
- 4-5 artichoke hearts, chopped
- 1 cup arugula
- 2 tbsp pesto
- 2 cups shredded cheese
- ½ tsp dried basil
- ½ tsp dried parsley
- ½ tsp dried oregano
- ½ tsp garlic salt

Note:
Dough can be frozen after rising. Just thaw and stretch, top, bake.

Directions

1. Mix warm water and molasses until dissolved. Add yeast and let sit until foamy (about 5 minutes).
2. Add flour and salt to the mixer/bowl and whisk together.
3. Add wet ingredients and olive oil to the flour mixture.
4. Knead on low with a dough hook for about 5 minutes until tacky and smooth.
5. Form into a ball and place in a lightly greased bowl.
6. Cover and let rise for about 1 hour (until doubled in size).
7. Preheat the oven to 500°F (if using pizza stone, preheat in oven).
8. Scatter a little flour or cornmeal on pizza stone or baking sheet.
9. Stretch dough to your desired shape and brush with olive oil.
10. (For crispier crust) bake dough (without topping) for 2 minutes.
11. Mix together chopped artichokes, herbs, shredded cheese and pesto.
12. Remove from the oven, top with arugula and cheese mixture and then bake for 7-9 minutes until the cheese is lightly browned and bubbly.
13. Slice and ENJOY!

Carb-licious Dinner & Sides

Pesto Artichoke Arugula Pizza
continued

Variations

- Adding herbs and grated Parmesan cheese to the dough adds a lovely boost of flavor!
- To make calzones, shape dough into a circle, fill half with toppings and cheese of choice, and fold the remaining half over. Press edges together to seal and cut 3 small slits on top of dough. Bake for 8-9 minutes until golden brown. Brush with olive oil and sprinkle with Parmesan.

Double Recipe
(2 large crusts, 3 medium, 4 small)

Crust

- 1 ½ cups warm water
- 1-2 tbsp molasses
- 4 ½ tsp dry active yeast
- 3 ½ cups flour
- 2 tsp salt
- 1 tbsp olive oil
- 2 tbsp Parmesan cheese (optional)

Toppings

- 8-10 artichoke hearts, chopped
- 2 cups arugula
- 4 tbsp pesto
- 4 cups shredded cheese
- 1 tsp dried basil
- 1 tsp dried parsley
- 1 tsp dried oregano
- 1 tsp garlic salt

Single Small Crust

Crust

- ½ cup and 2 tbsp warm water
- 1 tsp molasses
- 1 ⅛ tsp dry active yeast
- 1 ¾ cup and 2 tbsp flour
- ½ tsp salt
- 1 ½ tsp olive oil
- 1 tsp grated Parmesan cheese (optional)

Toppings

- 2-3 artichoke hearts, chopped
- ½ cup arugula
- 1 tbsp pesto
- 1 cup shredded cheese
- ¼ tsp dried basil
- ¼ tsp dried parsley
- ¼ tsp dried oregano
- ¼ tsp garlic salt

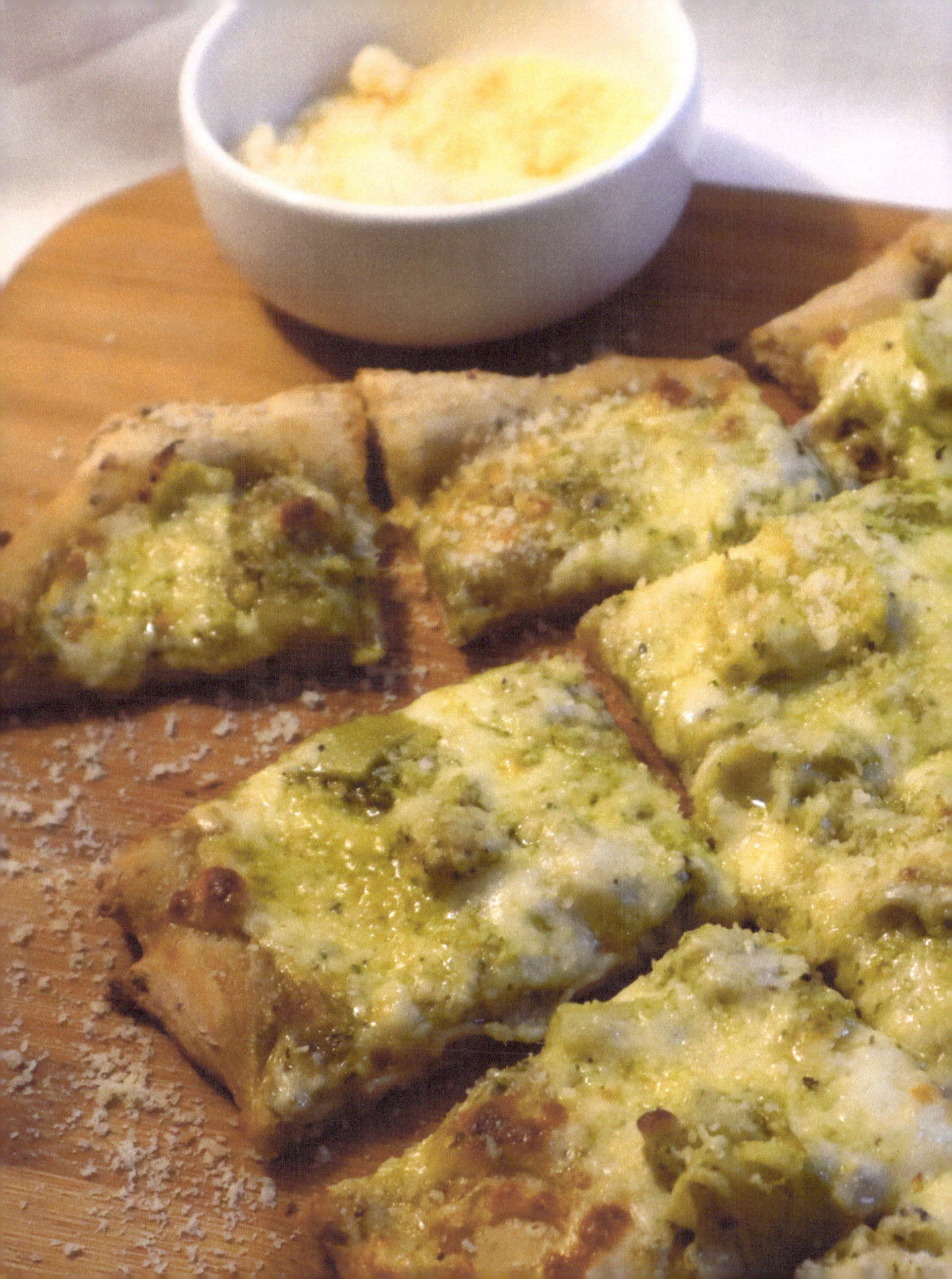

Avocado, Egg & Spinach Grilled Cheese

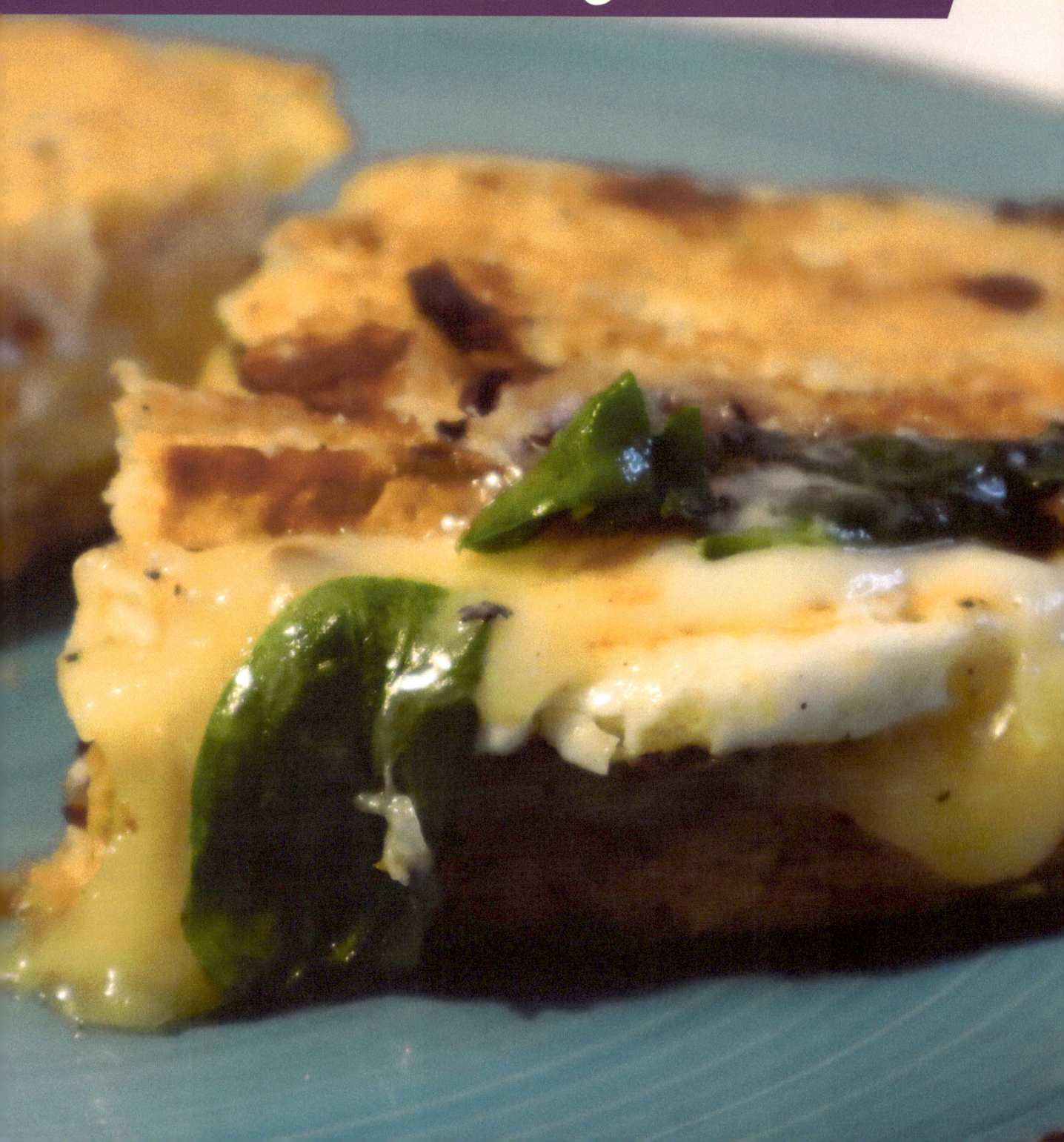

Grilled cheese is the best comfort food, in my opinion. While I still love your basic grilled cheese made with squishy white bread and cheese slices, this upgraded version is tastiness in every comforting, cheesy bite. Enjoy when you're feeling blue, irritated AF, hormonal, or riding the waves of grief. Or when you just want something simple and delicious.

Serving: 2 sandwiches

Prep Time: 5 minutes

Bake Time: 15 minutes

Ingredients

- 4 slices of bread (sourdough is excellent)
- ½ avocado
- 3-4 eggs, fried or scrambled
- 3-4 slices cheddar cheese
- Handful of spinach
- 1-2 tbsp butter
- Salt & pepper to taste

Directions

1. Fry or scramble 3-4 eggs, use salt and pepper to taste.
2. For an extra crispy sandwich, lightly toast bread before adding fillings.
3. Layer avocado, half the cheese, eggs, remaining cheese, and spinach between each pair of bread.
4. Butter outer sides of each sandwich and grill both sides on low-medium heat until medium brown and cheese is melty.
5. Cut in half and enjoy!

Variations

- Add a dash of lime juice to avocado for added zest.
- Substitute spinach for arugula or preferred greens.
- Substitute preferred cheese.
- Substitute pesto for avocado.

Double Recipe (4 sandwiches)

- 8 slices of bread (sourdough is excellent)
- 1 avocado
- 6-8 eggs, fried or scrambled
- 6-8 slices cheddar cheese
- 2 handfuls of spinach
- 2-4 tbsp butter
- Salt & pepper to taste

Single Serve (1 sandwich)

- 2 slices of bread (sourdough is excellent)
- ¼ avocado
- 1-2 eggs, fried or scrambled
- 2-3 slices cheddar cheese
- Handful of spinach
- 1 tbsp butter
- Salt & pepper to taste

Pesto Tortellini Mac & Cheese

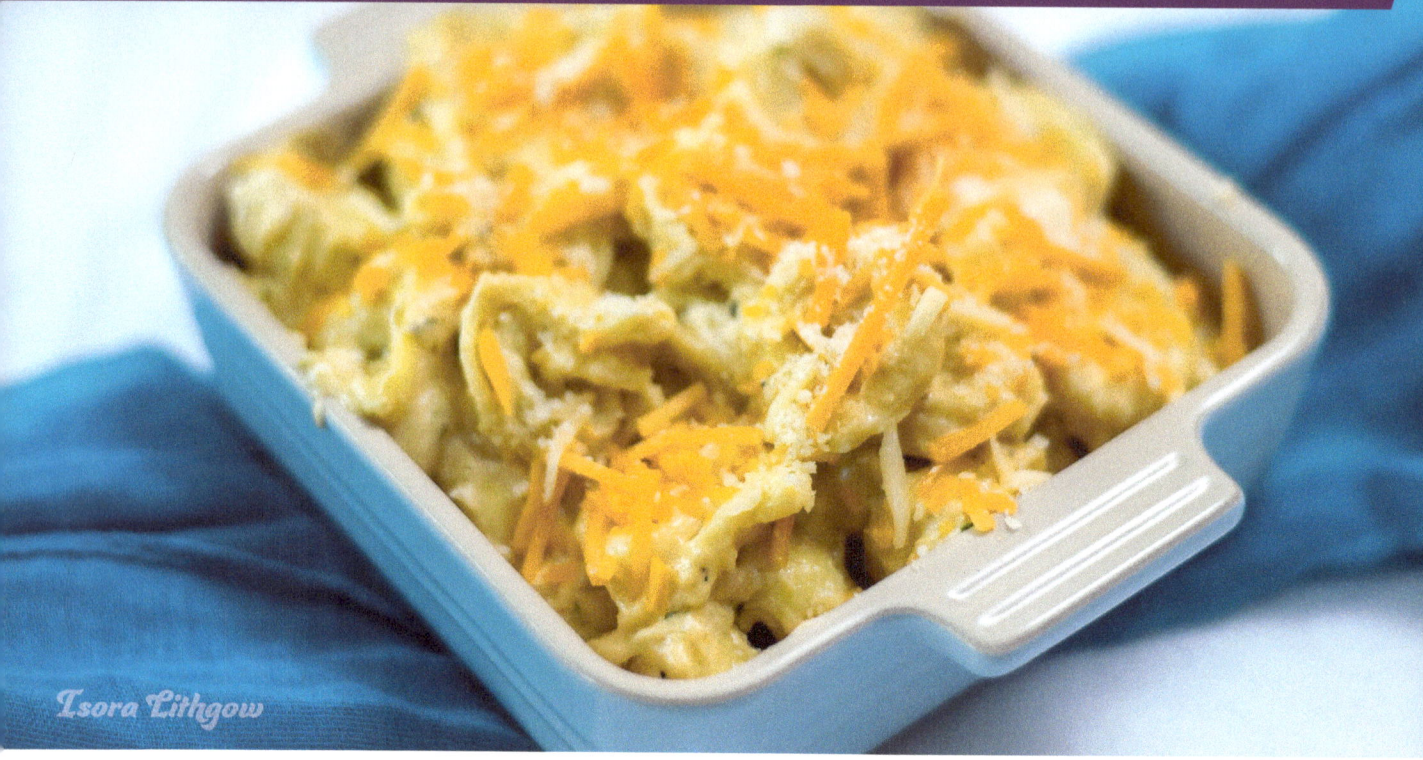

Isora Lithgow

Think traditional mac & cheese but a thousand times more decadent. Extra cheesy, a hint of pesto, and yummy tortellini make for mouth-watering bites that'll make you go back for more. Rich, savory, and made for warming the soul on cold, wintery nights. It's hard to go wrong with mac & cheese and this couldn't be more right.

Serving: 2 people

Prep Time: 5 minutes

Bake Time: 10-15 minutes

Ingredients

- 2 tbsp butter
- 1 tbsp flour
- 1 ½ cups milk
- 3 cups tortellini *(or pasta of choice)*
- ½ tsp Kosher salt
- 3 tbsp pesto
- 1 cup shredded cheese
- 2 tbsp cream cheese
- ¼ cup grated Parmesan cheese
- Herbs to taste (parsley, basil, garlic, etc.) (I generally use ½ to 1 tsp each for dried herbs.)

Directions

1. Set pot of water to boil for pasta.
2. In a saucepan or stock pot, put butter, milk, flour, salt, pesto, cream cheese, Parmesan cheese, and half the shredded cheese. Heat on medium until boiling and beginning to thicken.
3. Once it starts to thicken, turn down heat and simmer while pasta cooks.
4. Once pasta has cooked at al dente, drain and set aside.
5. Add remaining shredded cheese to sauce and stir until melted.
6. Add desired herbs to sauce.
7. Toss pasta in sauce until well coated.
8. Serve hot and topped with an extra sprinkle of Parmesan cheese. Garnish with toasted panko crumbs for a bit of crunch.
9. Enjoy!

Variations

- Swap cream cheese for creamy ricotta or goat cheese.
- Add lightly roasted veggies for extra flavor and fun.
- To turn into baked mac & cheese: after tossing pasta in sauce, put in an oven safe dish and sprinkle with extra shredded cheese and toasted panko crumbs. Bake for 20 minutes or until the cheese is melted and bubbly.

Note:

Can use any pasta you prefer, tortellini just gives an extra feel of decadence!

Freeze in a freezer safe container for several months or store in the fridge for several days.

Double Recipe (3-4 people)

- 4 tbsp butter
- 2 tbsp flour
- 3 cups milk
- 6 cups tortellini *(or pasta of choice)*
- 1 tsp Kosher salt
- 4 tbsp pesto
- 2 cups shredded cheese
- 4 tbsp cream cheese
- ½ cup grated Parmesan cheese
- Herbs to taste (parsley, basil, garlic, etc.) (I generally use 1 to 1 ½ tsp each for dried herbs.)

Single Serve (1 person)

- 1 tbsp butter
- ½ tbsp flour
- ½ cup milk
- 1 ½ cups tortellini *(or pasta of choice)*
- ¼ tsp Kosher salt
- 1 ½ tbsp pesto
- ½ cup shredded cheese
- 1 tbsp cream cheese
- ⅛ cup grated Parmesan cheese
- Herbs to taste (parsley, basil, garlic, etc.) (I generally use ½ to 1 tsp each for dried herbs.)

Carb-licious Dinner & Sides

Khachapuri (Georgian Cheese Bread)

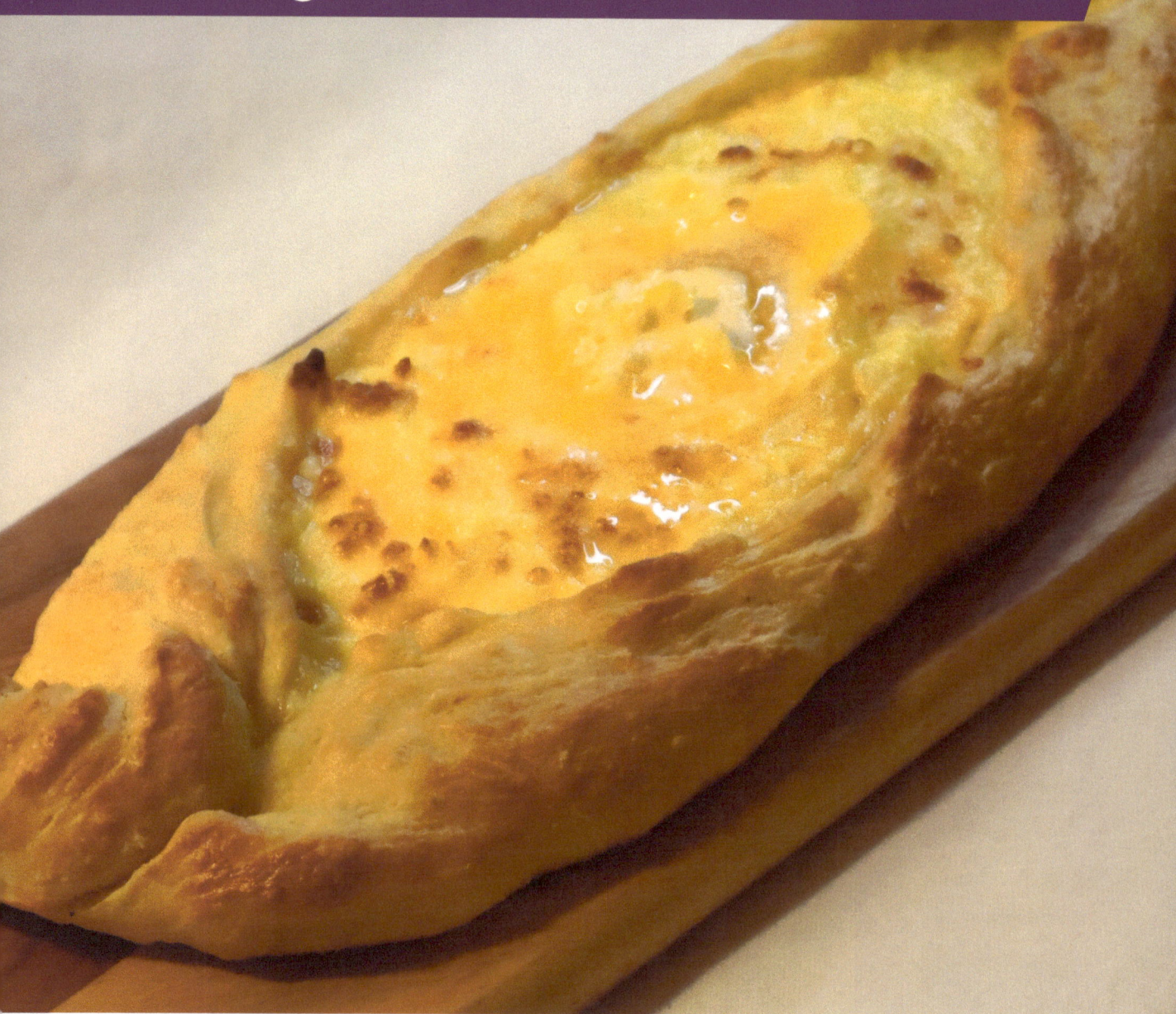

It's a bread boat filled with egg and cheese. Perfect for breakfast, lunch or dinner. Tear off chunks of bread and swirl in eggy goodness. I dare you to try not going back for just one more bite. And one more.

Serving:
1-2 people (1 Khachapuri)

Prep Time:
1 hour, 15 minutes

Bake Time:
15 minutes

Carb-licious Dinner & Sides

Ingredients

Dough
- ¾ cup + 2 tbsp bread flour
- ½ tsp instant yeast
- ¼ tsp salt
- ¼ cup water, room temp
- 2 tbsp slightly warmed milk
- ¾ tsp olive oil
- 1 egg white

Filling
- 1 + ½ cup mozzarella cheese, divided (freshly grated or shredded)
- 4 oz feta cheese, crumbled
- 1 whole egg
- Splash of feta brine or milk
- 1 egg yolk
- 1 tbsp butter, room temp

Directions

1. Preheat the oven to 500°F.

Dough
2. Combine flour, yeast, and salt in a bowl.
3. Make well in the middle. Add water, milk, and olive oil.
4. Work flour into liquid until it forms a shaggy dough.
5. Knead by hand or with a dough hook until smooth (about 5 minutes).
6. Place in a lightly greased bowl and cover with plastic or towel for about 1 hour, or until doubled in size.
7. Once doubled, punch down and form into a round. Keep covered and let rest for 20 minutes.

Filling
8. Combine cheeses and whole egg. Add feta brine or milk to form a sort of paste.

Shaping
9. Roll or stretch dough to form a 10-12" oval/rectangle (approximate) about ¼ inch thick.
10. Spread cheese mixture on dough, leaving ½ inch around the edge.
11. Fold the long edge of dough slightly over the cheese mixture on both sides. Pinch narrow ends together and twist twice to seal, making boat shape.
12. Add extra cheese to top and brush dough with egg white wash.
13. Cook until the cheese mixture is hot and bubbly and the dough is golden brown, about 8-9 minutes.
14. Remove, make a well in the center. Add egg yolk and cook for an additional 2-3 minutes.
15. Remove and add tbsp of butter. While still hot, swirl cheese, yolk, and butter together with a fork.
16. Eat and enjoy!

Khachapuri (Georgian Cheese Bread)
continued

Variations
- Add herbs of choice to the cheese mixture.
- Add artichoke hearts, asparagus, tomatoes, etc.
- Add pesto.

Double Recipe
(2-4 people, 2 Khachapuri)

Dough
- 1 ¾ cups bread flour
- 1 tsp instant yeast
- ½ tsp salt
- ½ cup water, room temp
- ¼ cup slightly warmed milk
- 1 ½ tsp olive oil
- 1 egg white

Filling
- 2 + 1 cup mozzarella cheese, divided (freshly grated or shredded)
- 8 oz feta cheese, crumbled
- 2 whole egg
- Splash of feta brine or milk
- 2 egg yolk
- 2 tbsp butter, room temp

Single Serve
(1 person, 1 small Khachapuri)

Dough
- ½ cup bread flour
- ¼ tsp instant yeast
- ⅛ tsp salt
- 2 tbsp water, room temp
- 1 tbsp slightly warmed milk
- ½ tsp olive oil
- 1 egg white

Filling
- ½ + ¼ cup mozzarella cheese, divided (freshly grated or shredded)
- 2 oz feta cheese, crumbled
- ½ whole egg
- Splash of feta brine or milk
- 1 egg yolk
- ½ tbsp butter, room temp

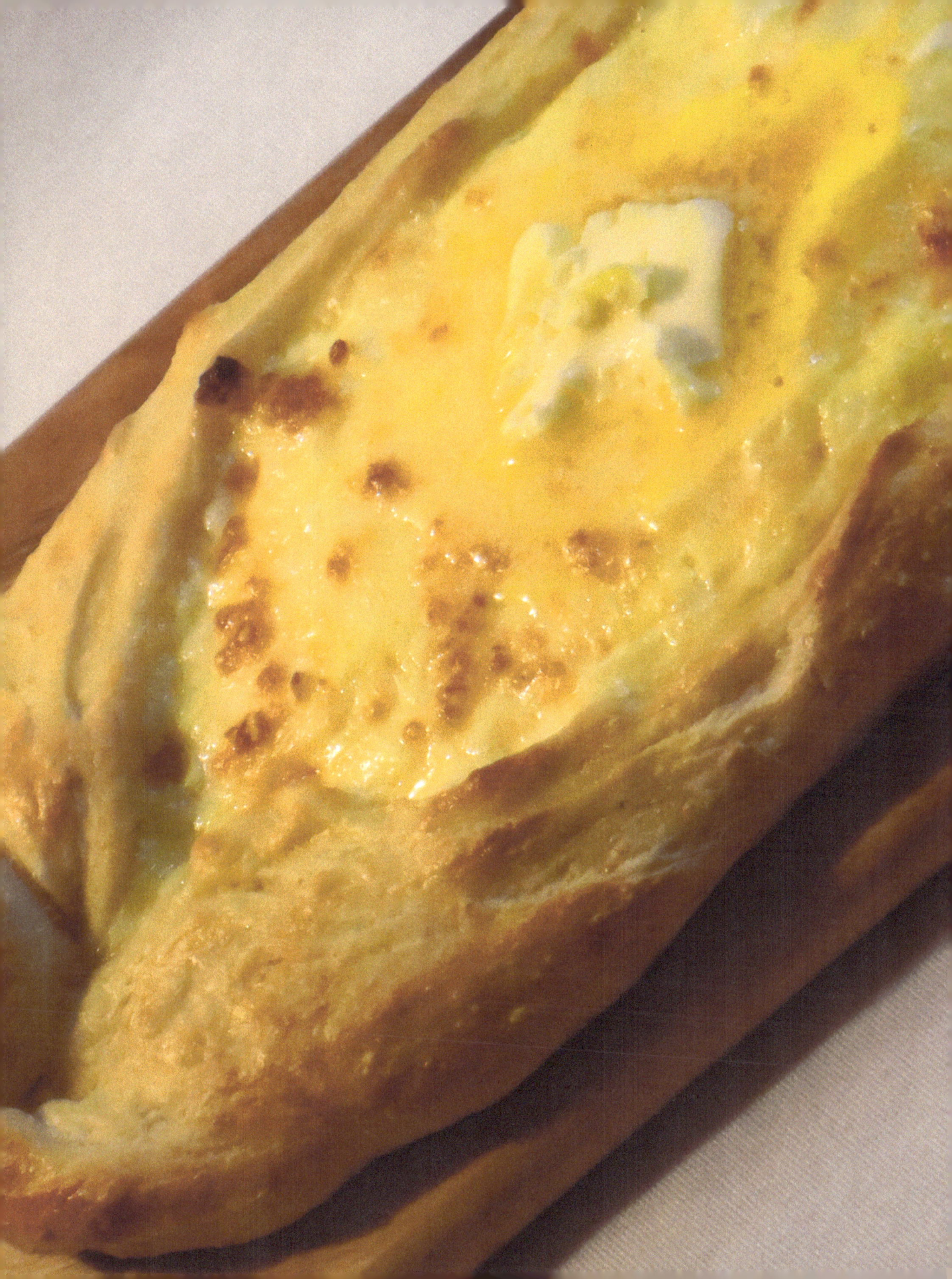

Rice & Veggie Bowl

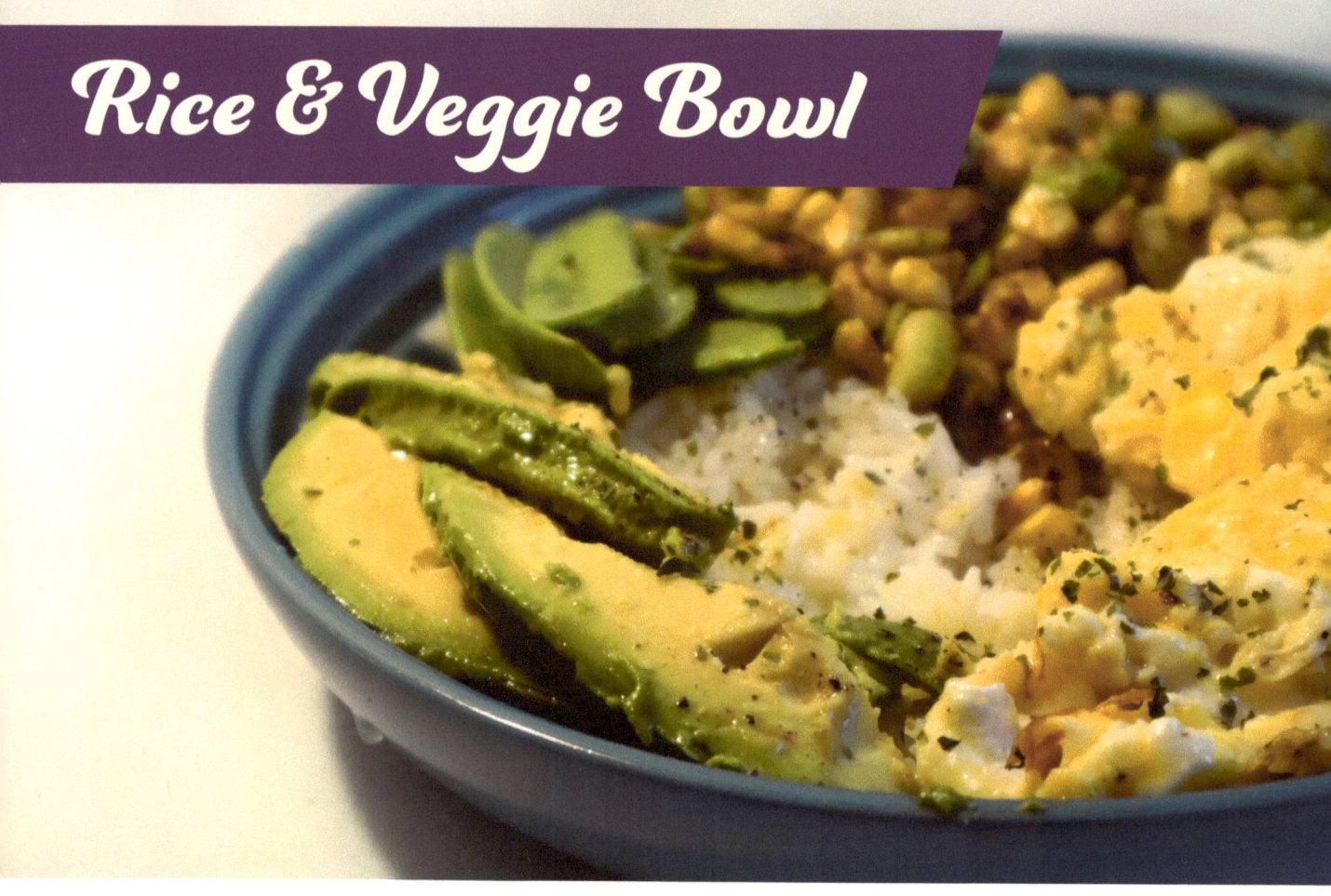

I love all-in-one meals, one bowl and it's got everything to fill up and satisfy—veggies, carbs, and protein. Simple flavors that together make a tasty bowl of yum for the belly. The little kick of lime is a MUST.

Serving:
2 bowls

Prep Time:
10 minutes

Bake Time:
30 minutes

Ingredients

- 1 ½ cups rice
- 2 cups water
- 1 tsp butter
- ⅓ cup corn
- ⅓ cup edamame
- Handful snow peas
- ½ avocado, sliced
- 3-4 eggs
- ⅓ cup shredded cheese
- Splash of milk
- 1 tsp olive oil
- 1 lime
- 1 tsp cilantro
- Salt & pepper to taste

Directions

1. Cook rice and butter in water over medium heat (or in a rice cooker), until water is absorbed and rice is soft.
2. Roast corn and edamame in a skillet with olive oil, salt and pepper until tender and lightly charred.
3. Scramble eggs with a splash of milk, adding shredded cheese for the last 30 seconds to a minute of cooking.
4. Slice ½ an avocado.
5. Plate rice, top with avocado, corn, edamame, snow peas, and eggs.
6. Add salt, pepper and cilantro to taste.
7. Squeeze lime over a bowl and enjoy!

Variations

- Can substitute any preferred veggies or whatever you have on hand.
- Mix cooked rice with pesto.
- Replace eggs with chicken or preferred meat and/or tofu.
- Substitute orzo or other pasta for rice.

Double Recipe (4 bowls)

- 3 cups dry rice
- 4 cups water
- 2 tsp butter
- ⅔ cup corn
- ⅔ cup edamame
- Large handful snow peas
- 1 avocado, sliced
- 6 eggs
- ½ cup shredded cheese
- ¼ cup milk
- 1 tsp olive oil
- 2 limes
- 2 tsp cilantro
- Salt & pepper to taste

Single Serve (1 bowl)

- ¾ cup dry rice
- 1 cup water
- ½ tsp butter
- ¼ cup corn
- ¼ cup edamame
- Handful snow peas
- ¼ avocado, sliced
- 2 eggs
- ¼ cup shredded cheese
- Splash of milk
- 1 tsp olive oil
- 1 lime
- ½ tsp cilantro
- Salt & pepper to taste

Carb-licious Dinner & Sides

Herby Roasted Potatoes

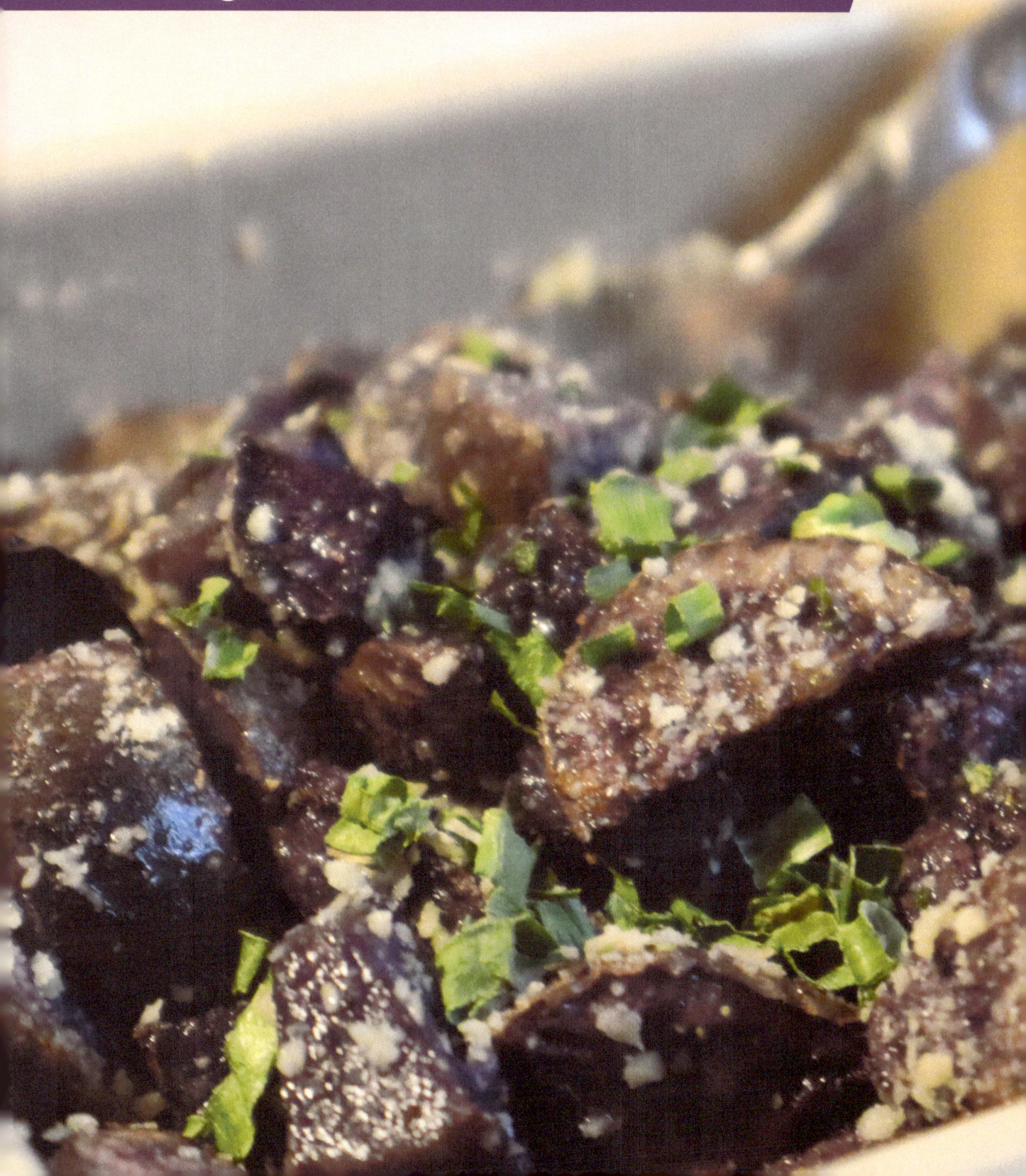

Tender, crisp bites of potato and bursts of herby flavors make a lovely accompaniment to any meal. I personally am a fan of using purple potatoes—they taste the same as your typical white potatoes but they make an extra pretty plate!

Serving:
4 people

Prep Time:
10 minutes

Bake Time:
20-25 minutes

Ingredients

- 3-4 large russet potatoes (or 8-9 fingerling potatoes), diced
- 2 tsp olive oil
- 1 tsp parsley
- 1 tsp thyme
- 1 tsp rosemary
- 1 ½ tsp garlic
- Salt & pepper to taste
- 2 tbsp grated Parmesan

Directions

1. Preheat the oven to 425°F.
2. Dice potatoes into bite sized pieces (about ½ in).
3. Toss potatoes with olive oil, herbs, and salt/pepper.
4. Spread in single layer on baking sheet and roast for about 20-25 minutes, turning about half way through, until easily pierced by fork and slight crispy on edges.
5. Toss with grated Parmesan and enjoy!

Variations

- Substitute for any preferred combination of herbs.
- Use purple or rainbow potatoes for a fun change.

Double Recipe (8 people)

- 6-9 large russet potatoes (or 15-17 fingerling potatoes), diced
- 4 tsp olive oil
- 2 tsp parsley
- 2 tsp thyme
- 2 tsp rosemary
- 3 tsp garlic
- Salt & pepper to taste
- 4 tbsp grated Parmesan

Single Serve (1 person)

- 1 large russet potato (or 4-5 fingerling potatoes), diced
- 1 tsp olive oil
- ½ tsp parsley
- ½ tsp thyme
- ½ tsp rosemary
- 1 tsp garlic
- Salt & pepper to taste
- 1 tbsp grated Parmesan

Creamy Mashed Potatoes

Another adaptation snagged from my mom's recipes! **(Seriously, she's a great cook. I'd try to talk her into making a cookbook but she never makes the same recipe twice!)** The cream cheese is a must for extra creamy and smooth potatoes. And, honestly, add butter, salt and cheese until your arteries cry and your taste buds dance. You won't regret it.

Serving:	Prep Time:	Bake Time:
4 people	15 minutes	25 minutes

Ingredients

- 4 large russet potatoes
- 4 oz cream cheese, softened
- 6 tbsp butter, softened
- ½ cup milk
- ½ cup shredded cheese of choice (cheddar, mozzarella, etc)
- 1 tsp parsley
- 1 tsp chives
- 1 tsp garlic salt
- Salt & pepper to taste

Directions

1. Cut and quarter potatoes and put in the pot. Cover with water and boil until tender.
2. Drain water and place potatoes in a large mixing bowl.
3. Add cubed cream cheese and butter, cheese, milk and herbs.
4. Mash with potato masher or fork until combined.
5. Add salt and pepper to taste.
6. Serve warm and enjoy!

Variations

- Peel potatoes prior to boiling if you prefer no skins.
- Substitute various herbs as desired.
- Add bacon bits or veggies.

Double Recipe (8 people)

- 8 large russet potatoes
- 8 oz cream cheese, softened
- 12 tbsp butter, softened
- 1 cup milk
- 1 cup shredded cheese of choice (cheddar, mozzarella, etc)
- 2 tsp parsley
- 2 tsp chives
- 2 tsp garlic salt
- Salt & pepper to taste

Single Serve (1 person)

- 1 large russet potato
- 1 oz cream cheese, softened
- 1 ½ tbsp butter, softened
- 2 tbsp milk
- ⅛ – ¼ cup shredded cheese of choice (cheddar, mozzarella, etc)
- ¼ tsp parsley
- ¼ tsp chives
- ¼ tsp garlic salt
- Salt & pepper to taste

Carb-licious Dinner & Sides

Cheesy Garlic Potato Skins

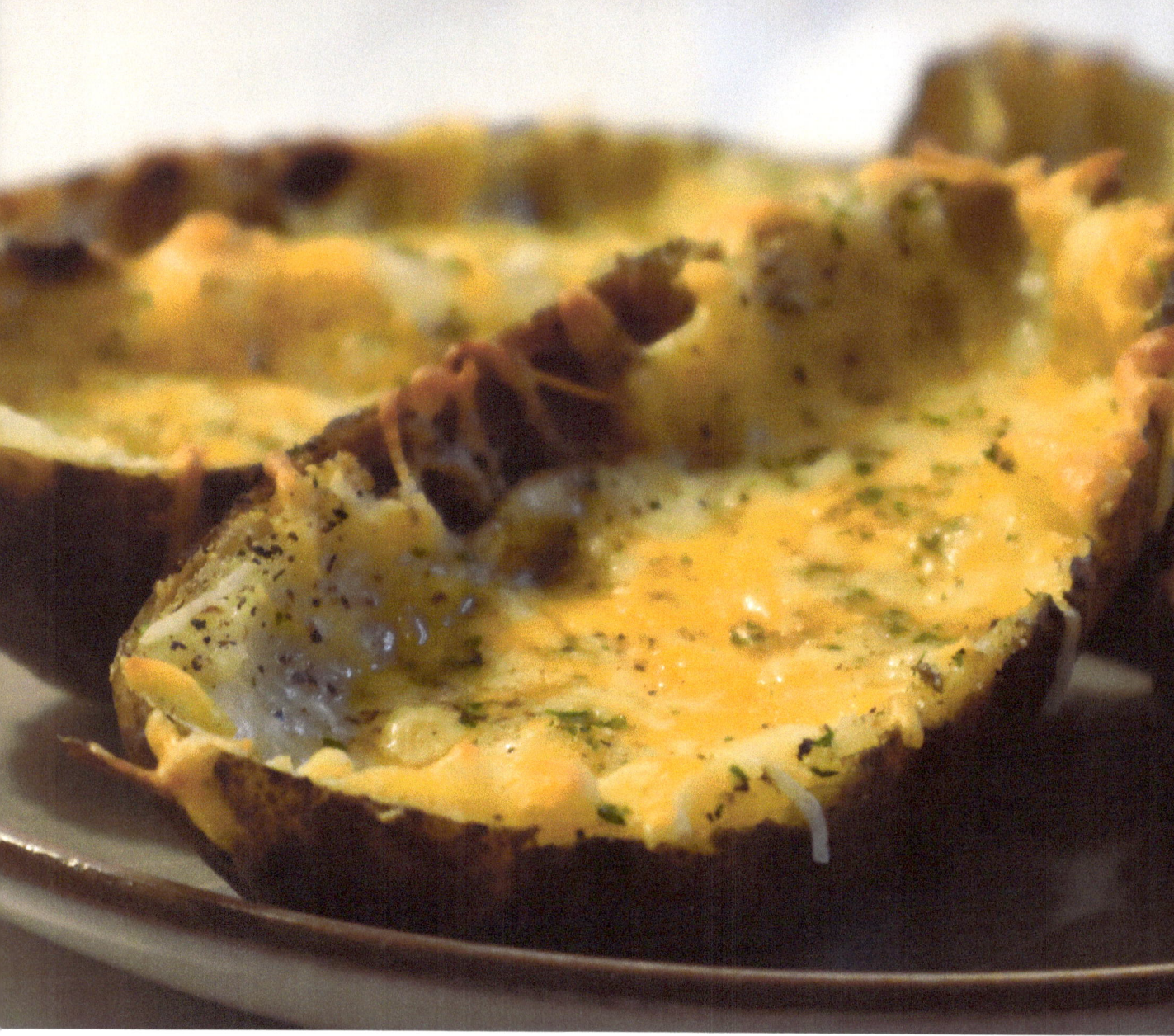

As you can see, I'm a fan of potatoes in their many versatile forms. I mean, how can you not love them? Potato skins are your favorite sport-watching, party appetizer, or satisfy the hungry kiddos, plate of munchies. Dip in sour cream, top with bacon (if you must), or enjoy as is. Wherever you enjoy them, your belly will be pleased.

Serving:
12 potato skins

Prep Time:
15-20 minutes

Bake Time:
1 hour, 15 minutes

Carb-licious Dinner & Sides

Ingredients

- 6 russet potatoes
- ½ – ¾ cup shredded cheese
- ½ tsp garlic salt
- 3 tbsp melted butter
- 1 tbsp chives (dry or fresh)
- Salt & pepper to taste
- Olive oil
- Optional: bacon bits

Directions

1. Preheat the oven to 400°F.
2. Rub potatoes with olive oil and salt/pepper before wrapping in aluminum foil.
3. Bake for about 1 hour or until they give slightly when squeezed.
4. Allow potatoes to cool until able to handle.
5. Cut potatoes in half and remove most of the inner flesh, leaving a thin layer with the skin. Arrange on a baking sheet.
6. Melt butter and mix with garlic salt.
7. Brush potato skins with butter mix.
8. Fill halves with shredded cheese and sprinkle with chives and salt/pepper. (Add bacon bits if desired.)
9. Return the baking sheet with potatoes to the oven and bake for about 10-15 minutes or until the cheese is melted and bubbly.
10. Cool for a few minutes and enjoy!

Note:
Can be prepared and frozen for future use, just thaw and warm in the oven.

Double Recipe (24 skins)

- 12 russet potatoes
- 1 cup shredded cheese
- 1 tsp garlic salt
- 6 tbsp melted butter
- 1-2 tbsp chives (dry or fresh)
- Salt & pepper to taste
- Olive oil
- Optional: bacon bits

Single Serve (6 skins)

- 3 russet potatoes
- ¼ – ⅓ cup shredded cheese
- ¼ tsp garlic salt
- 2 tbsp melted butter
- ½ tbsp chives (dry or fresh)
- Salt & pepper to taste
- Olive oil
- Optional: bacon bits

Chocolate Peanut Butter Layer Cake

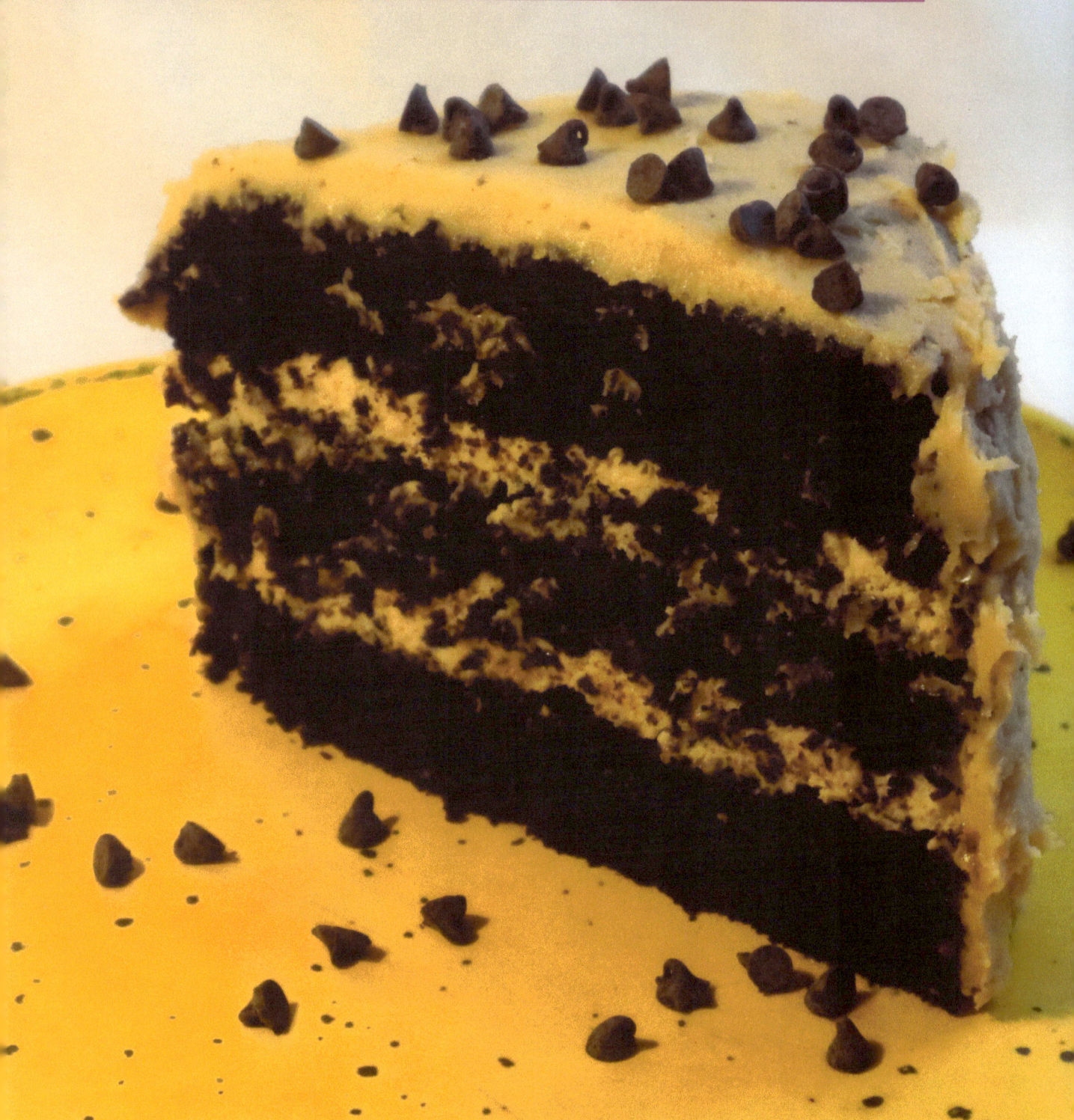

It's chocolate and peanut butter. Layered together. Basically, it's sheer bliss on a plate. Need I say more?

Serving:
One 9-inch cake

Prep Time:
2 hours

Bake Time:
1 hour

Ingredients

Cake

- 2 ¼ cups flour
- 1 ½ cups sugar
- ⅔ cup dark cocoa powder
- ¾ tsp salt
- ½ tsp espresso powder (optional)
- 1 ½ tsp baking soda
- 2 ¼ tsp vanilla
- 1 ½ tbsp white vinegar
- ⅓ + ¼ cup vegetable oil
- 1 ½ cups water

Mousse

- 1 tsp + ⅛ tsp powdered gelatin
- 1 ½ tbsp water
- 9 ounces peanut butter chips
- 2 ¼ cups heavy whipping cream
- ¼ cup powdered sugar

Frosting

- ¼ cup + 2 tbsp softened butter
- 6 oz cream cheese (brick-style)
- 1 ½ tsp vanilla
- ¼ tsp salt
- 3 cups powdered sugar
- ½ – ¾ cup creamy peanut butter

Directions

Cake

1. Preheat the oven to 350°F. Lightly grease a 8 or 9-inch cake pan.
2. Mix dry ingredients together in a medium bowl.
3. Mix vanilla, vinegar, vegetable oil, and water in a separate bowl.
4. Pour wet ingredients into a bowl of dry ingredients, stirring until completely combined.
5. Pour ⅓ batter into the cake pan.
6. Bake for 15-20 minutes, until a toothpick inserted in the center of the cake comes out clean. Cool cake completely before removing from pan. Repeat for all 3 layers.

Mousse

7. In small bowl, sprinkle the gelatin over water, let stand for 5 minutes.
8. Place peanut butter chips in medium bowl.
9. Heat ¾ cup of heavy cream until it comes to a full boil.
10. Add gelatin to heavy cream and whisk until dissolved.
11. Pour cream over peanut butter chips and let sit for a minute.
12. Whisk until peanut butter is melted and smooth. Set aside to cool about 5 minutes.
13. Whisk remaining heavy cream at high speed until it begins to thicken.

Chocolate Peanut Butter Layer Cake

continued

14. Add powdered sugar and whip until stiff peaks form.
15. Fold ⅓ whipped cream into peanut butter mixture until well combined.
16. Add remaining whipped cream and fold.
17. Chill in the fridge for 1 hour to semi-set.
18. Pipe between layers of cooled cake.
19. Chill before frosting.

Frosting

20. Cream butter, peanut butter, and cream cheese until smooth and lump free.
21. Add vanilla and salt and mix well.
22. Gradually add powdered sugar until completely combined.
23. Add a thin crumb coat of frosting to cooled cake.
24. Chill cake in the fridge for 1 hour.
25. Add the final coat of frosting to cake.
26. Enjoy!

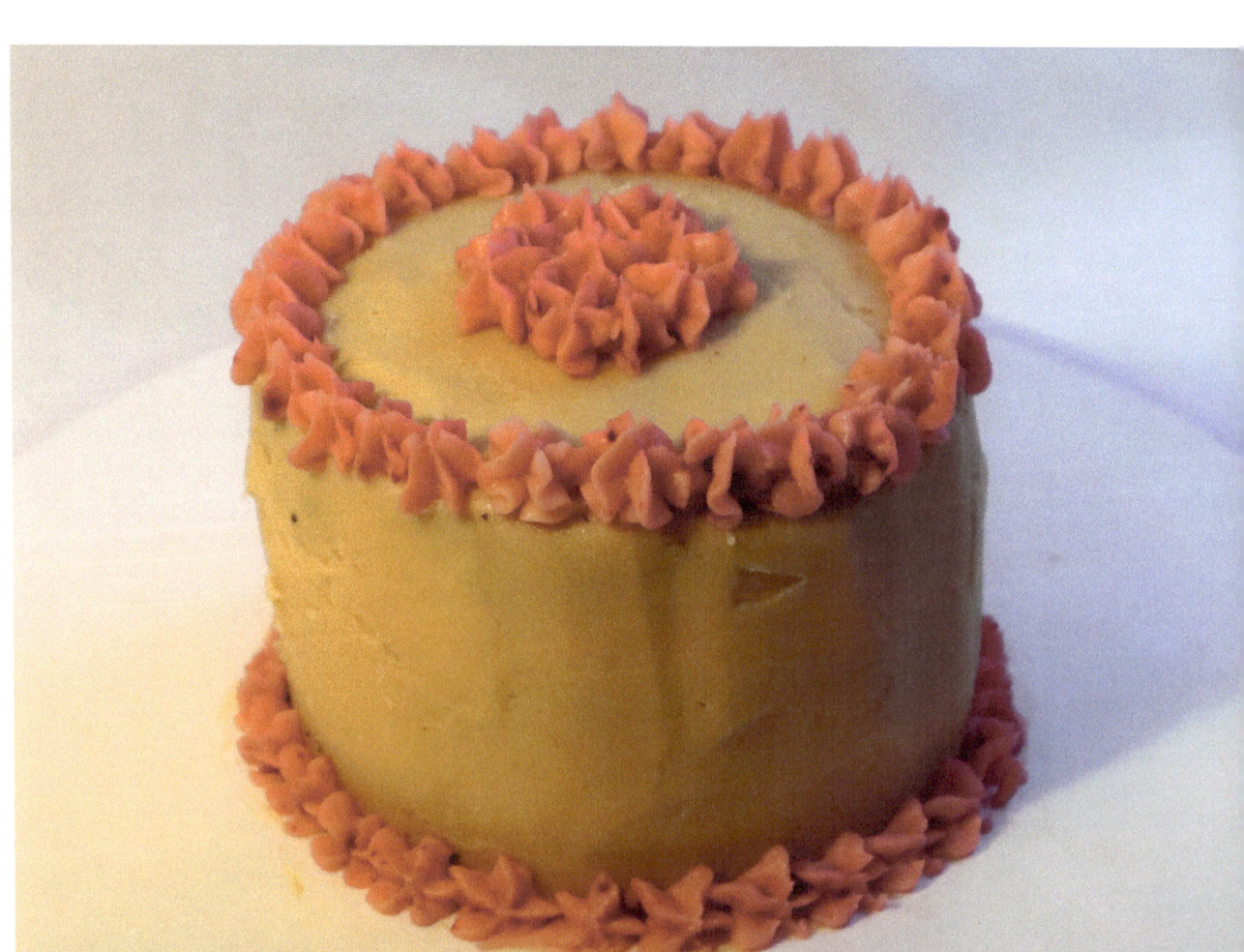

Variations

- Can substitute chocolate, vanilla, raspberry, strawberry, etc. for peanut butter.

> **Note:**
> Chill cake for about an hour prior to cutting to reduce crumbs.
>
> I find it helpful to bake the cakes a day ahead of time and do layers and frosting the next day.

Double Recipe
(two 9-inch cakes)

Cake

- 4 ½ cups flour
- 3 cups sugar
- 1 ⅓ cups dark cocoa powder
- 1 ½ tsp salt
- 1 tsp espresso powder (optional)
- 3 tsp baking soda
- 4 ½ tsp vanilla
- 3 tbsp white vinegar
- ⅔ + ½ cup vegetable oil
- 3 cups water

Mousse

- 2 tsp + ¼ tsp powdered gelatin
- 3 tbsp water
- 18 ounces peanut butter chips
- 4 ½ cups heavy whipping cream
- ½ cup powdered sugar

Frosting

- ¾ cup softened butter
- 12 oz cream cheese (brick-style)
- 3 tsp vanilla
- ½ tsp salt
- 6 cups powdered sugar
- 1 – 1 ½ cups creamy peanut butter

Single Serve
(one 4-inch cake)

Cake

- 1 ⅛ cup flour
- ¾ cup sugar
- ⅓ cup dark cocoa powder
- ½ tsp salt
- ¼ tsp espresso powder (optional)
- ¾ tsp baking soda
- 1 ⅛ tsp vanilla
- ¾ tbsp white vinegar
- ½ cup + 1 tbsp vegetable oil
- ¾ cup water

Mousse

- ½ tsp powdered gelatin
- ¾ tbsp water
- 4 ½ ounces peanut butter chips
- 1 ⅛ cups heavy whipping cream
- ⅛ cup powdered sugar

Frosting

- 3 tbsp softened butter
- 3 oz cream cheese (brick-style)
- ¾ tsp vanilla
- ⅛ tsp salt
- 1 ½ cups powdered sugar
- ¼ – ½ cup creamy peanut butter

Creamy Vanilla Cheesecake

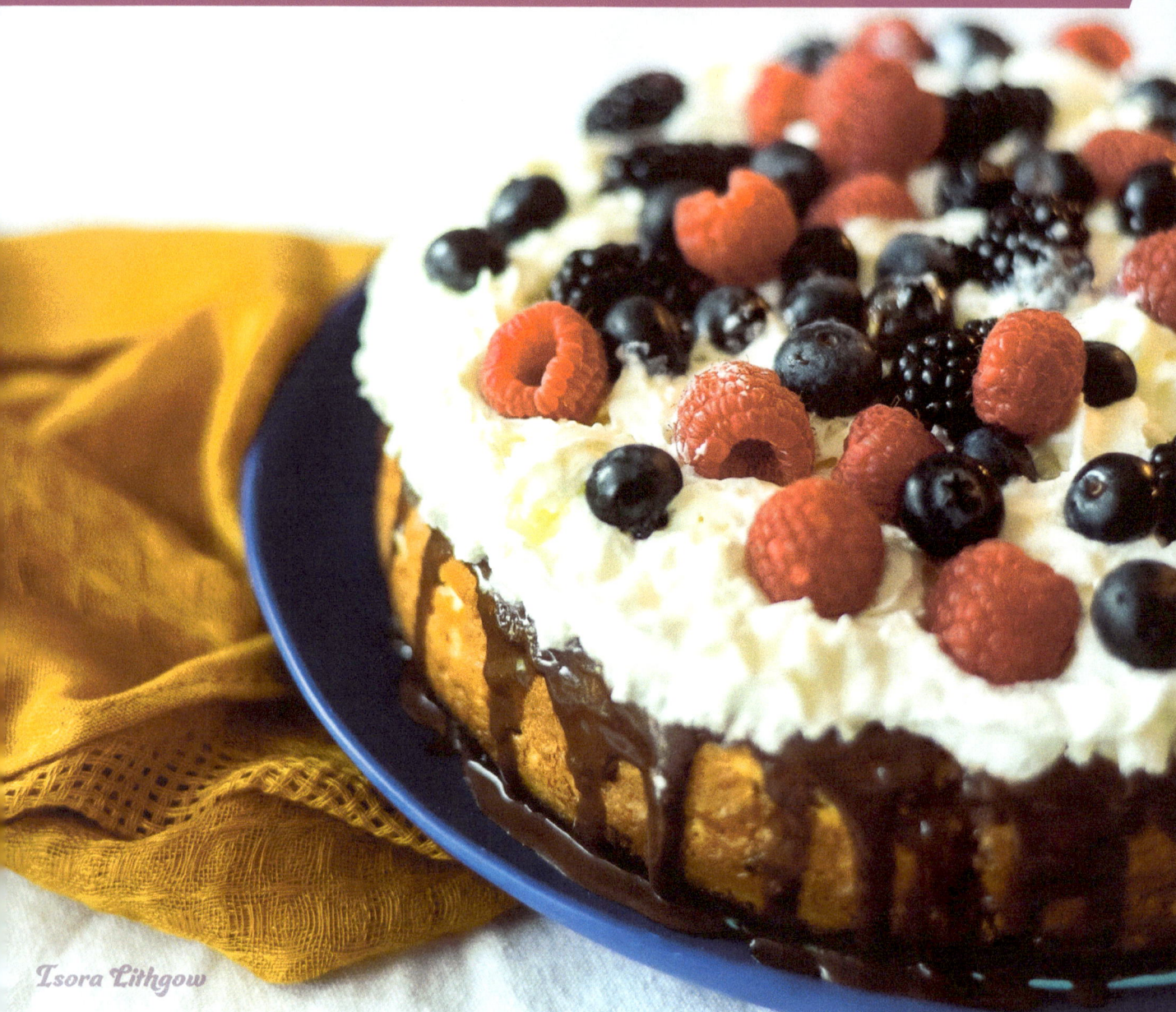

Isora Lithgow

Years ago in college I found the original recipe that this cheesecake evolved out of on the back of an Oreo pie crust package. It made a regular appearance on girls night with my college buddy, Natalie. We ate a lot of cheesecake back in the day! This version is even better, creamier, and more irresistible than it's college tested origin cake. Use a good quality Greek vanilla yogurt for the most amazing result!

Serving:
One 9-inch cake

Prep Time:
20 minutes

Bake Time:
1 – 1.5 hours

Ingredients

Crust
- 20 crushed whole Oreos
- ¼ cup powdered sugar
- 4 tbsp melted butter

Filling
- 2 packages softened cream cheese (16 oz)
- ⅔ cup sugar
- 3 egg whites
- 2 tsp vanilla
- 2 cups vanilla yogurt
- 2 tbsp flour

> **Note:**
> Can use premade crust for ease if desired.

Directions

1. Preheat the oven to 375°F. Lightly grease a 9-inch springform pan.

Crust
2. Use a food processor to crush/crumble Oreos with powdered sugar (or classic rolling pin and ziplock bag if no food processor).
3. Add melted butter, mixing until evenly crumbly. Press moist crumbs into the bottom and slightly up the sides of the greased pan.
4. Place the pan on a baking sheet and bake for 15 minutes. Remove from the oven and set aside.

Filling
5. Reduce oven heat to 325°F.
6. Beat together cream cheese until smooth.
7. Add sugar, egg whites, and vanilla and beat until smooth (about 2 minutes).
8. Beat in yogurt and flour on low speed until smooth.
9. Pour batter into the crust. Keep the pan on a baking sheet for ease of getting in and out of the oven.
10. Bake for 50-60 minutes until the toothpick comes out of the outside edge cleanly. Center may not be set but this is fine.
11. Turn off the oven, crack the door open and let the cake cool in the oven for 30 minutes.
12. Remove from oven and let cool 15 minutes.
13. Cover and refrigerate until ready to serve.
14. Enjoy!

Creamy Vanilla Cheesecake
continued

Variations

- Replace Oreos with graham crackers for crust.
- Drizzle with melted chocolate and dust with powdered sugar (or raspberry/strawberry powder) or garnish with fresh fruit.
- Drizzle with caramel and garnish with nuts.
- Drizzle with fruit sauce and dust with powdered sugar.
- Coat with melted chocolate and add whipped cream.

Double Recipe
(two 9-inch cakes)

Crust

- 40 crushed whole Oreos
- ½ cup powdered sugar
- 8 tbsp melted butter

Filling

- 4 packages softened cream cheese (32 oz)
- 1 ⅓ cups sugar
- 6 egg whites
- 4 tsp vanilla
- 4 cups vanilla yogurt
- ¼ cup flour

Single Serve
(one 4-inch cake)

Crust

- 10 crushed whole Oreos
- 2 tbsp powdered sugar
- 2 tbsp melted butter

Filling

- 1 packages softened cream cheese (8 oz)
- ⅓ cup sugar
- 2 egg whites
- 1 tsp vanilla
- 1 cup vanilla yogurt
- 1 tbsp flour

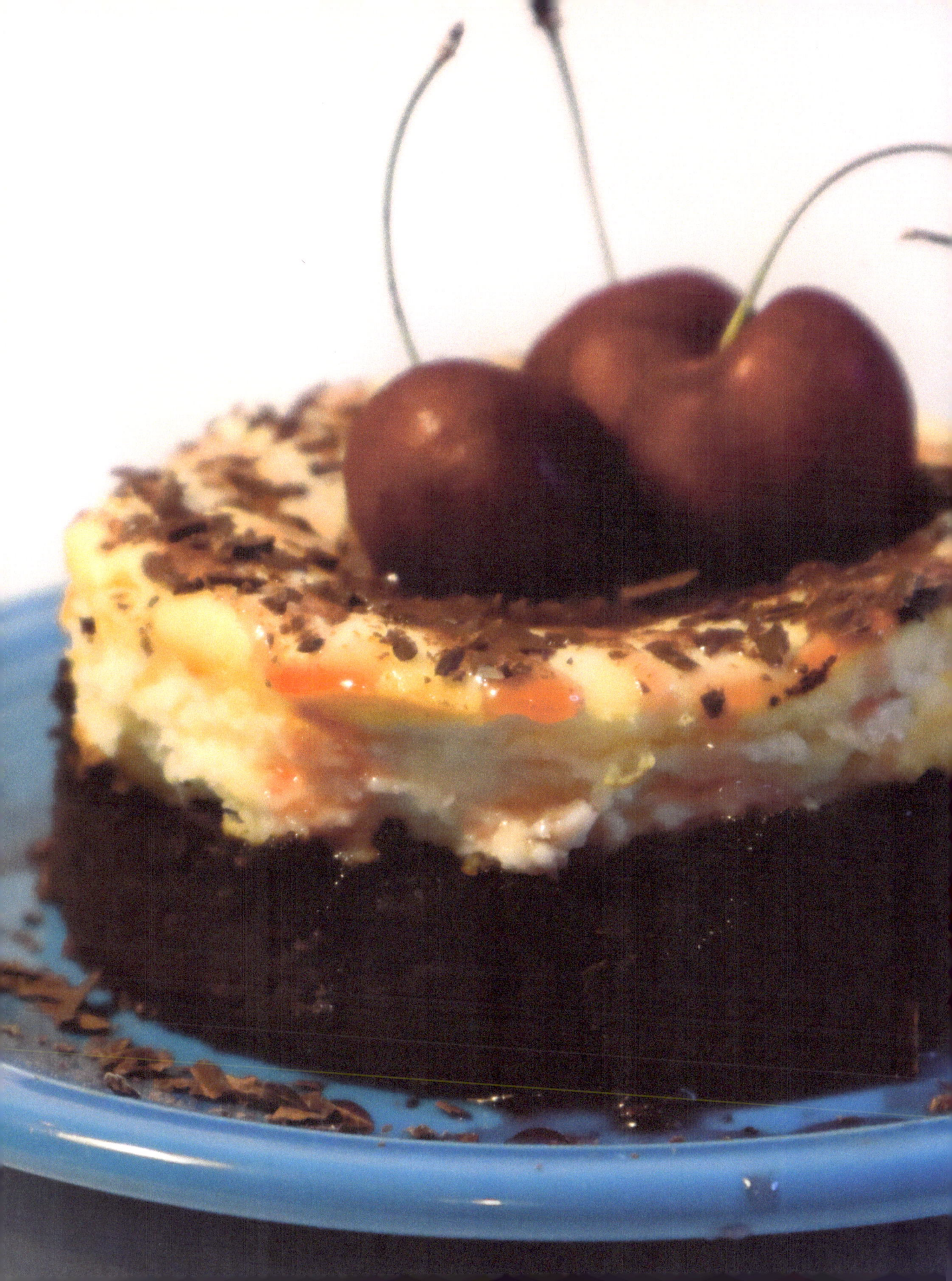

Chocolate Mousse Cake

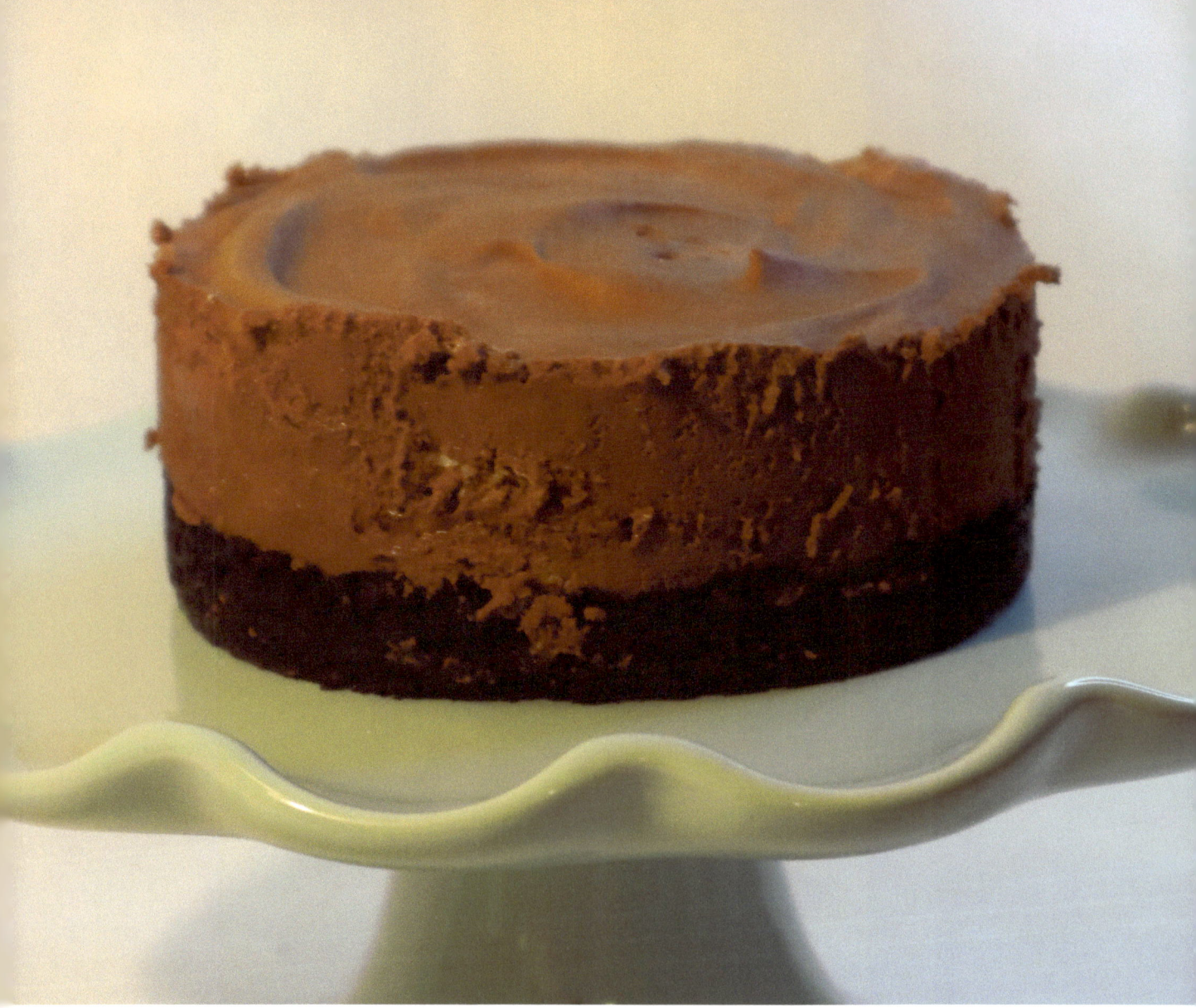

My favorite bakery, Mirabelles, in Burlington, VT makes the most amazing Raspberry Chocolate Mousse Cake that I adore. It's what inspired me to try to make a mousse cake of my own (although this cake is absolutely nothing like theirs!). If I'd known how easy it was to make mousse, I'd have started making it years ago. A fudgy chocolate brownie bottom covered with rich dark chocolate mousse—seriously, how can it be anything but amazing?!

Serving:
One 9-inch cake

Prep Time:
30 minutes

Bake Time:
25-30 minutes

Ingredients

Brownie Crust

- 1 stick (8 tbsp) softened butter
- ¾ cup semi sweet chocolate chips
- ⅓ cup dark chocolate chips
- ¾ cup sugar
- 1 tbsp vanilla
- ½ tsp coffee granules
- 2 large eggs, room temp
- ¼ cup flour
- ⅓ cup cocoa powder
- ½ tsp baking powder

Mousse

- 2 tsp + ¼ tsp powdered gelatin
- 3 tbsp water
- 18 ounces semisweet chocolate chips
- 4 ½ cups heavy whipping cream
- ½ cup powdered sugar

Directions

Brownie Crust

1. Preheat the oven to 350°F. Line a 9-inch pan with parchment paper.
2. Melt together butter, semi sweet, and dark chocolate chips until smooth.
3. Stir in sugar, vanilla, and coffee.
4. Mix eggs into chocolate mix.
5. Add flour, cocoa powder, and baking powder and mix until just combined.
6. Spread mixture into the baking pan.
7. Bake for 25-30 minutes or until just set.
8. Set aside to cool completely.

Mousse

9. In small bowl, sprinkle the gelatin over water, let stand for 5 minutes.
10. Place chocolate chips in medium bowl.
11. Heat ¾ cup of heavy cream until it comes to a full boil.
12. Add gelatin to heavy cream and whisk until dissolved.
13. Pour cream over chocolate chips and let sit for a minute.
14. Whisk until chocolate is melted and smooth. Set aside to cool about 5 minutes.
15. Whisk remaining heavy cream at high speed until it begins to thicken.
16. Add powdered sugar and whip until stiff peaks form.
17. Fold ⅓ whipped cream into chocolate mixture until well combined.
18. Add remaining whipped cream and fold.
19. Spoon chocolate mousse over brownie (use a pan at least 4 inches tall) and put in fridge until firm (2-3 hours).

Chocolate Mousse Cake

continued

Variations

- Substitute raspberry, vanilla, strawberry, etc. mousse for chocolate.
- Layer several different kinds of mousse on top of each other.

Note:

To cut smoothly, run knife under hot water and wipe dry just before cutting.

Can be stored in airtight container in fridge for several days.

Double Recipe (two 9-inch cakes)

Brownie Crust

- 2 sticks (16 tbsp) softened butter
- 1 ½ cups semi sweet chocolate chips
- ⅔ cup dark chocolate chips
- 1 ½ cups sugar
- 2 tbsp vanilla
- 1 tsp coffee granules
- 4 large eggs, room temp
- ½ cup flour
- ⅔ cup cocoa powder
- 1 tsp baking powder

Mousse

- 4 ½ tsp powdered gelatin
- 6 tbsp water
- 36 ounces semi sweet chocolate chips
- 9 cups heavy whipping cream
- 1 cup powdered sugar

Single Serve (one 4-inch cake)

Brownie Crust

- ½ stick (4 tbsp) softened butter
- ¼ cup + 2 tbsp semi sweet chocolate chips
- ¼ cup dark chocolate chips
- ¼ cup + 2 tbsp sugar
- ½ tbsp vanilla
- ¼ tsp coffee granules
- 1 large egg, room temp
- 2 tbsp flour
- ¼ cup cocoa powder
- ¼ tsp baking powder

Mousse

- 1 tsp + ¼ tsp powdered gelatin
- 1 ½ tbsp water
- 9 ounces semi sweet chocolate chips
- 2 ¼ cups heavy whipping cream
- ¼ cup powdered sugar

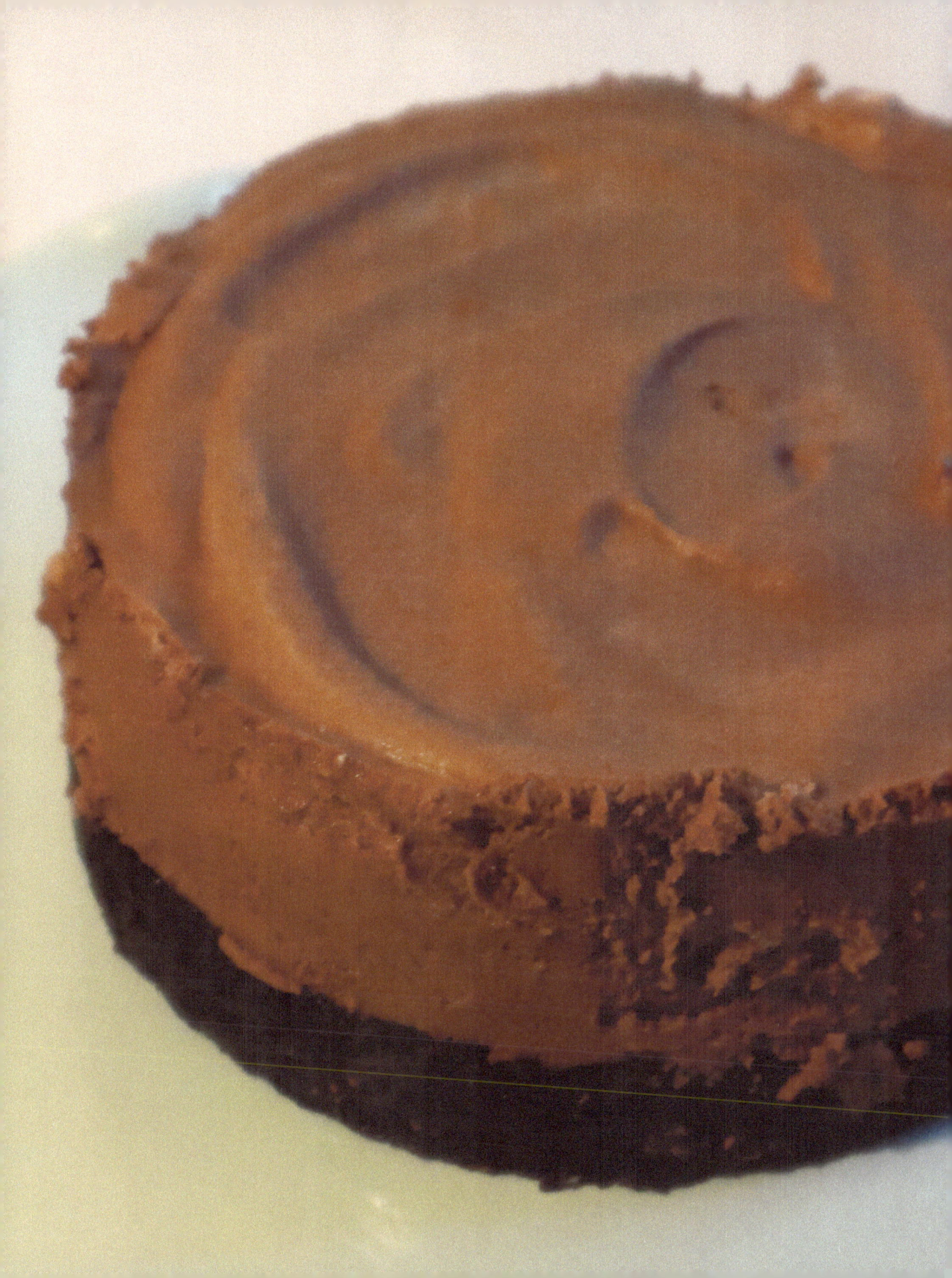

Cinnamon Cake

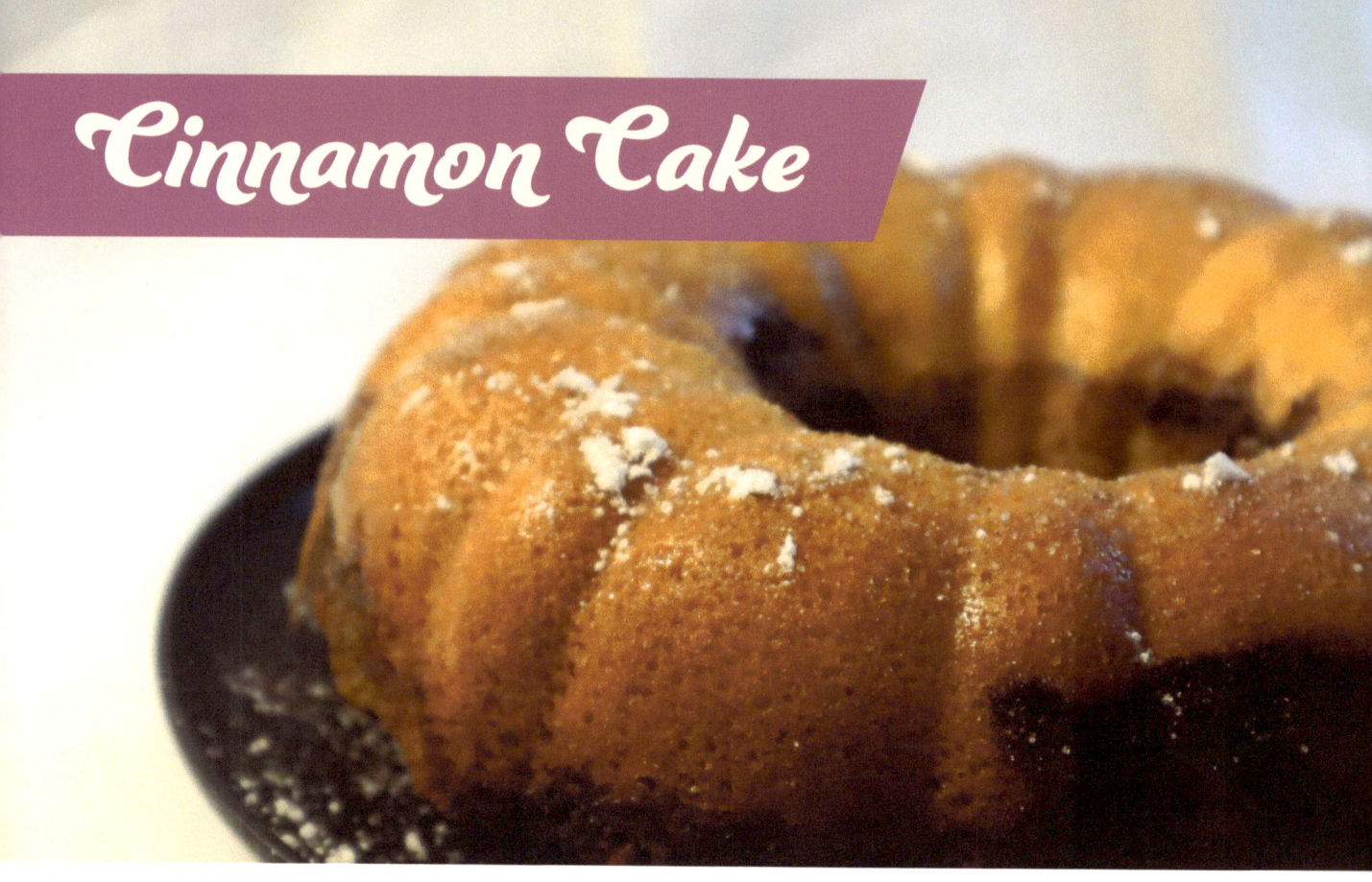

Cinnamon might just be my favorite spice. On the rare occasion I decide to expand my horizons for something sweet that doesn't involve chocolate, cinnamon is top of the list. And this cinnamon cake is moist, bursting with cinnamon, and close enough to a coffee cake (in my opinion) to use as an excuse to enjoy it for breakfast. Then again, food rules are silly so forget the excuse. You want cake for breakfast? Go ahead and enjoy, friend!

Serving:
10-12 people

Prep Time:
1 hour

Bake Time:
40-45 minutes

Ingredients

- 3 tbsp brown sugar
- 1 ½ tbsp cinnamon
- ½ tsp nutmeg
- 6 tbsp softened butter
- 1 cup sugar
- 3 eggs
- 1 ¾ cups + 2 tbsp flour
- 2 tbsp cornstarch
- 1 tsp baking powder
- ½ tsp baking soda
- ¼ tsp salt
- 1 cup sour milk (1 tbsp white vinegar and top off with 1 cup milk. Let sit for 10-15 minutes)
- 2 tsp vanilla

Directions

1. Preheat the oven to 325°F.
2. In a small bowl, mix together brown sugar, cinnamon and nutmeg.
3. In a large bowl, cream butter and sugar, then add eggs, one at a time, and vanilla and beat until fluffy.
4. In a medium bowl, shift together flour and cornstarch, then mix in baking powder, baking soda, and salt.
5. Add dry ingredients, alternating with sour milk, ending with sour milk. Mix well.
6. Spoon ⅓ of batter into a greased baking pan. Sprinkle half of the cinnamon mixture. Spoon another ⅓ of batter on top before adding remaining cinnamon mixture. Finish the remaining batter.
7. Bake for approximately 40-45 minutes or until a toothpick comes out clean and dry. Remove and let cool.

Variations

- For a sweeter option, drizzle cooled cake with icing.

Double Recipe (20-24 people)

- 6 tbsp brown sugar
- 3 tbsp cinnamon
- 1 tsp nutmeg
- 12 tbsp softened butter
- 2 cups sugar
- 6 eggs
- 3 ¾ cups flour
- 4 tbsp cornstarch
- 2 tsp baking powder
- 1 tsp baking soda
- ½ tsp salt
- 2 cups sour milk (2 tbsp white vinegar and top off with 2 cups milk. Let sit for 10-15 minutes.)
- 4 tsp vanilla

Single Serve (4-6 people)

- 1 ½ tbsp brown sugar
- ¾ tbsp cinnamon
- ¼ tsp nutmeg
- 3 tbsp softened butter
- ½ cup sugar
- 1 ½ eggs
- ¾ cup + 3 tbsp flour
- 1 tbsp cornstarch
- ½ tsp baking powder
- ¼ tsp baking soda
- ⅛ tsp salt
- ½ cup sour milk (½ tbsp white vinegar and top off with ½ cup milk. Let sit for 10-15 minutes.)
- 1 tsp vanilla

Rich Chocolate Cheesecake

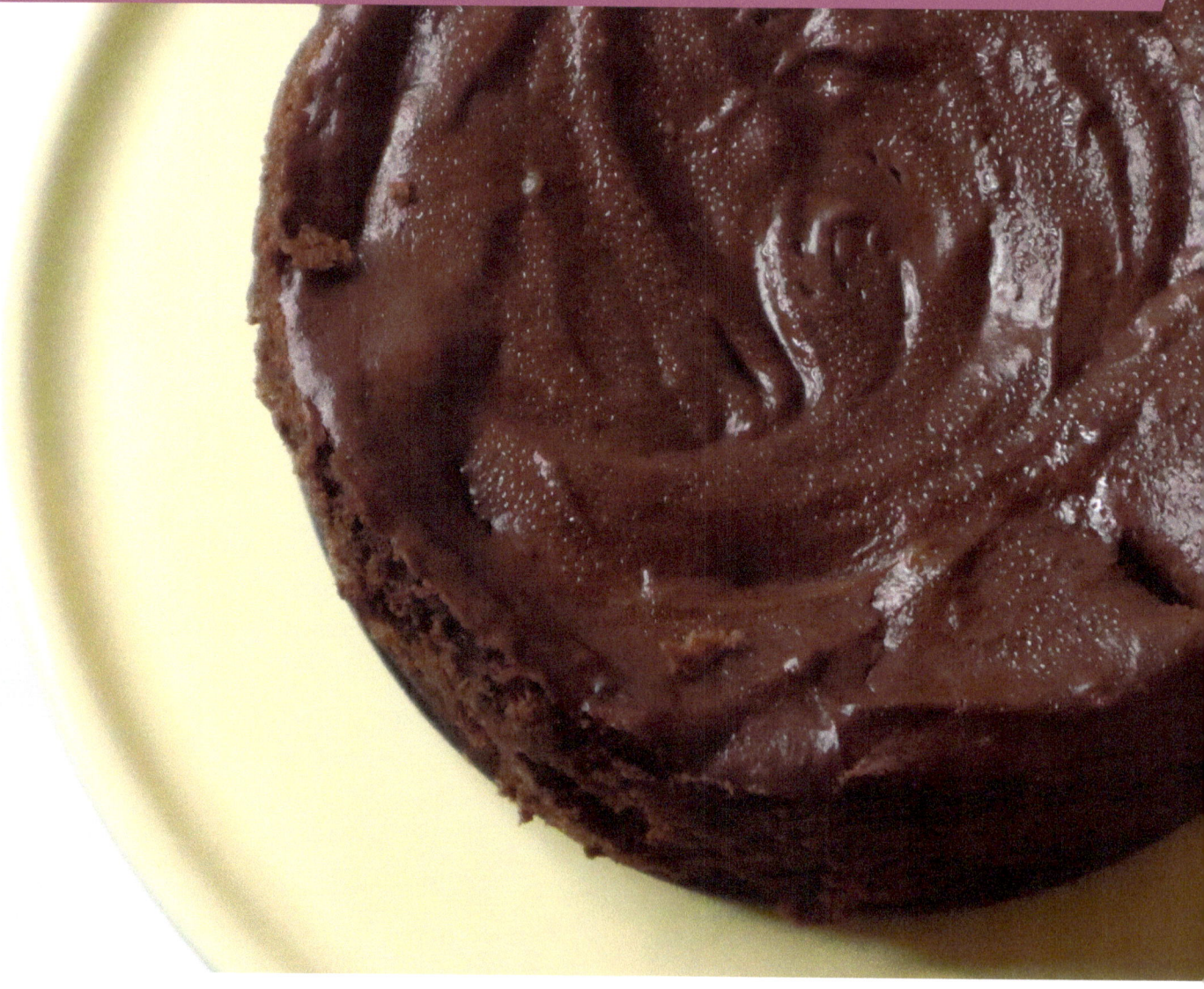

If I could live inside a cake, it would be this one. Rich, creamy, deeply chocolatey cheesecake with crushed Oreos for a crust—need I say more? One bite and you'll want to move in too. Take me home to you, baby.

Serving:
One 9-inch cake

Prep Time:
20 minutes

Bake Time:
1 – 1.5 hours

Ingredients

Crust
- 20 crushed whole Oreos
- ¼ cup powdered sugar
- 4 tbsp melted butter

Filling
- ½ cup milk
- 1 ½ cups semisweet chocolate chips
- ½ cup dark chocolate chips
- ½ tsp espresso powder
- 3 packages of softened cream cheese (8 oz each)
- 1 cup sugar
- 4 large eggs, room temp
- 1 ½ tsp vanilla
- 2 tbsp flour

Note:
Can use all semisweet or dark chocolate chips as preferred.

Coffee granules are optional—coffee just enhances chocolate flavor.

Can use premade crust for ease if desired.

Oreos can be replaced with graham crackers for crust if desired.

Directions

1. Preheat the oven to 375°F. Lightly grease a 9-inch springform pan.

Crust
2. Use a food processor to crush/crumble Oreos with powdered sugar (or classic rolling pin and ziplock bag if no food processor).
3. Add melted butter, mixing until evenly crumbly. Press moist crumbs into the bottom and slightly up sides of the greased pan.
4. Place the pan on a baking sheet and bake for 15 minutes. Remove from the oven and set aside.

Filling
5. Reduce oven heat to 350°F.
6. Heat milk, semisweet, and dark chocolate chips and stir until fully melted and smooth.
7. Remove from heat, add espresso powder and set aside.
8. Beat together cream cheese and sugar at low speed until thoroughly combined and smooth.
9. Add eggs one at a time, beating to combine after each one.
10. Stir in vanilla and then flour.
11. Add melted chocolate, beating slowly and thoroughly until combined and smooth.
12. Pour batter into the crust. Keep the pan on a baking sheet for ease of getting in and out of the oven.
13. Bake for 45-50 minutes until a toothpick comes out of the outside edge cleanly. Center may not be set but this is fine.
14. Turn off the oven, crack the door open and allow the cake to cool in the oven for 1 hour.
15. When completely cool, cover and refrigerate until ready to serve.
16. Garnish with extra Oreo crumbs or whipped cream and enjoy!

Cakes

Rich Chocolate Cheesecake
continued

Double Recipe
(two 9-inch cakes)

Crust
- 40 crushed whole Oreos
- ½ cup powdered sugar
- 8 tbsp melted butter

Filling
- 1 cup milk
- 3 cups semisweet chocolate chips
- 1 cup dark chocolate chips
- 1 tsp espresso powder
- 6 packages of softened cream cheese (8 oz each)
- 2 cups sugar
- 8 large eggs, room temp
- 3 tsp vanilla
- ¼ cup flour

Single Serve
(One 4-inch cake)

Crust
- 10 crushed whole Oreos
- 2 tbsp powdered sugar
- 2 tbsp melted butter

Filling
- ¼ cup milk
- ¾ cups semisweet chocolate chips
- ¼ cup dark chocolate chips
- ¼ tsp espresso powder
- 1 ½ packages of softened cream cheese (12 oz total)
- ½ cup sugar
- 2 large eggs, room temp
- 1 tsp vanilla
- 1 tbsp flour

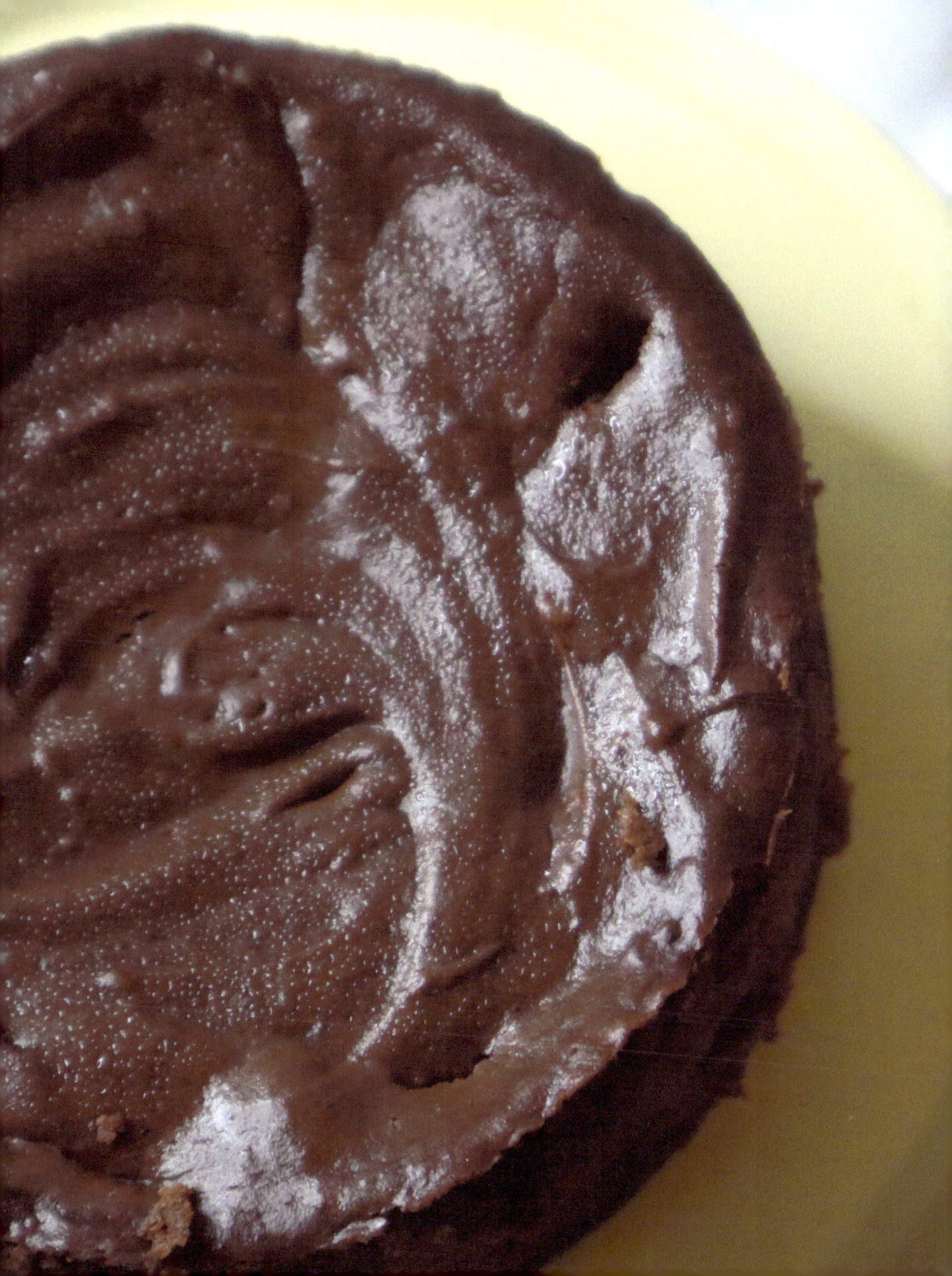

Vanilla Raspberry Layer Cake

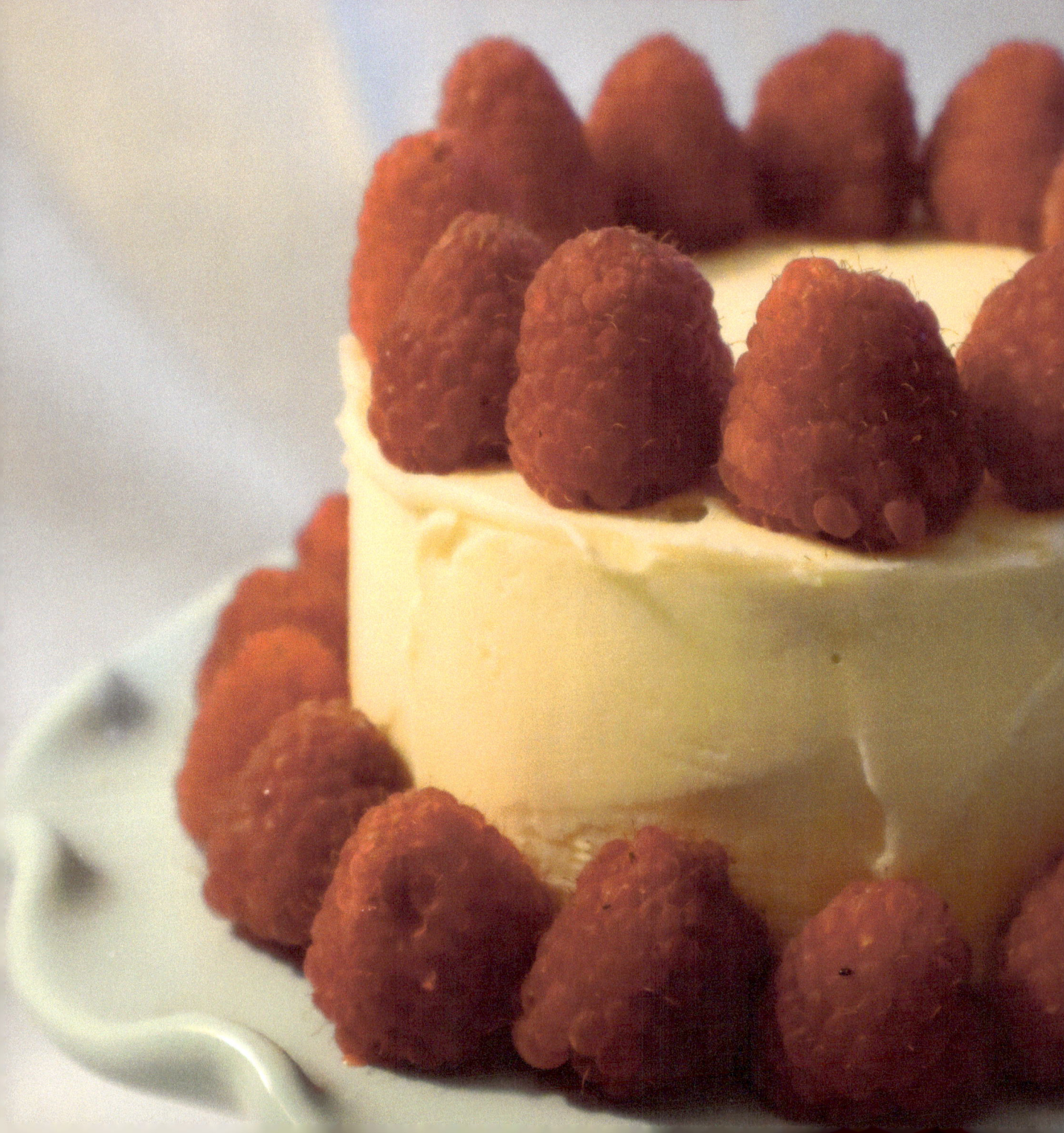

Normally, I'm alllll about raspberries with chocolate. Offer me anything raspberry + chocolate and I won't say no. So, I strayed a bit from my taste bud comfort zone by swapping chocolate for it's less intense cousin, vanilla. Light vanilla cake layered with fluffy raspberry mousse and wrapped in raspberry cream cheese frosting? Yes, please.

Serving:
One 9-inch cake

Prep Time:
50 minutes

Bake Time:
40 minutes

Ingredients

Cake

- 1 ¾ cups + 2 tbsp flour
- 2 tbsp cornstarch
- ¾ tsp salt
- 1 ½ tsp baking powder
- ½ tsp baking soda
- ¾ cup + 2 tbsp water
- ½ vegetable oil
- ¾ cup sugar
- 4 ½ tsp white vinegar
- 1 ½ tbsp vanilla
- ½ tsp almond extract

Raspberry Mousse

- ½ cup raspberries, frozen
- ¼ cup sugar
- 1 tbsp powdered sugar
- 1 ½ tbsp milk
- 1 ¼ cups whipping cream
- 1 ½ tsp powdered gelatin

Raspberry Cream Cheese Frosting

- ¼ cup softened butter
- 4 oz cream cheese (brick-style)
- 1 tsp vanilla
- ⅛ tsp salt
- 2 cups powdered sugar
- 3 tbsp powdered freeze dried raspberries

Directions

Cake

1. Preheat the oven to 350°F.
2. Whisk together flour and cornstarch.
3. Whisk in salt, baking soda, and baking powder.
4. In a separate bowl, whisk together water, vegetable oil, sugar, vinegar, vanilla, and almond extract.
5. Add wet ingredients to dry and stir to combine.
6. Grease 9-inch cake pan and pour in batter.
7. Bake for 30-35 minutes until the toothpick comes out clean.
8. Remove from the oven and let cool.
9. Once completely cool, cut the rounded top off. Then cut into two even layers.

> **Note:**
> I sometimes freeze the cake for one night before cutting it into layers. I find it makes it somewhat easier to divide.

Vanilla Raspberry Layer Cake

continued

Mousse

10. In small bowl, sprinkle gelatin over water and let sit for 5 minutes.
11. Puree frozen raspberries.
12. Heat raspberry puree with sugar and milk on the stove until just beginning to simmer.
13. Whisk in gelatin until dissolved.
14. Strain through a fine mesh strainer to remove pulp and seeds.
15. Store pulp and seeds for use in other recipes.
16. Whip remaining heavy cream on high until it begins to thicken.
17. Add powdered sugar and whip until stiff peaks form.
18. Fold 1/3 whipped cream into raspberry juice until well combined.
19. Fold in remaining whipped cream.
20. Cool fridge for 2-3 hours to set.

Frosting

21. Cream butter and cream cheese until smooth and lump free.
22. Add vanilla and salt and mix well.
23. Mix powdered sugar and powdered raspberry together.
24. Gradually add powdered sugar mixture until completely combined.
25. Frost completely cooled the cake.

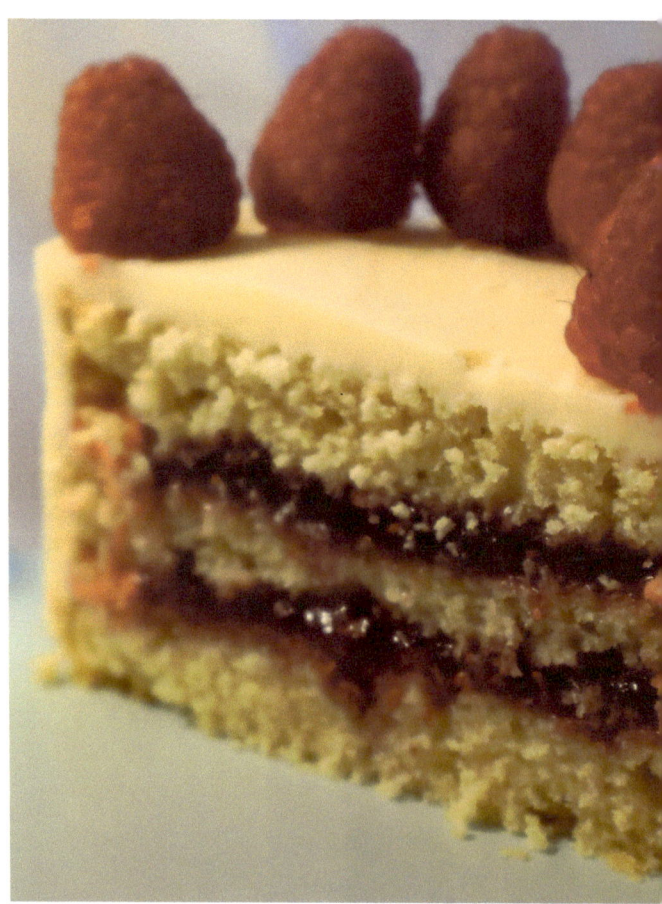

> **Note:**
> A crumb coat between each layer helps prevent the mousse from soaking into the cake.

Variations

- Substitute choice of fruit for raspberries or chocolate or peanut butter.
- Add fresh raspberries to mousse between layers.
- Dust top with leftover raspberry powder and/or add fresh raspberries.

Double Recipe (two 9-inch cakes)

Cake
- 3 ¾ cups flour
- 4 tbsp cornstarch
- 1 ½ tsp salt
- 3 tsp baking powder
- 1 tsp baking soda
- 1 ¾ cups water
- 1 cup vegetable oil
- 1 ½ cups sugar
- 3 tbsp white vinegar
- 3 tbsp vanilla
- 1 tsp almond extract

Raspberry Mousse
- 1 cup raspberries, frozen
- ½ cup sugar
- 2 tbsp powdered sugar
- 3 tbsp milk
- 2 ½ cups whipping cream
- 3 tsp powdered gelatin

Raspberry Cream Cheese Frosting
- ½ cup softened butter
- 8 oz cream cheese (brick-style)
- 2 tsp vanilla
- ¼ tsp salt
- 4 cups powdered sugar
- 6 tbsp powdered freeze dried raspberries

Single Serve (one 4-inch cake)

Cake
- ¾ cups + 2 ½ tbsp flour
- 1 tbsp cornstarch
- ¼ tsp salt
- ¾ tsp baking powder
- ¼ tsp baking soda
- ¼ cup + 2 ½ tbsp water
- ¼ vegetable oil
- 3 tbsp sugar
- 2 ¼ tsp white vinegar
- ¾ tbsp vanilla
- ¼ tsp almond extract

Raspberry Mousse
- ¼ cup raspberries, frozen
- ⅛ cup sugar
- ½ tbsp powdered sugar
- ¾ tbsp milk
- ½ cup + 2 tbsp whipping cream
- ¾ tsp powdered gelatin

Raspberry Cream Cheese Frosting
- 2 tbsp softened butter
- 2 oz cream cheese (brick-style)
- ½ tsp vanilla
- Pinch of salt
- 1 cup powdered sugar
- 1 ½ tbsp powdered freeze dried raspberries

Decadently Chocolate Brownies

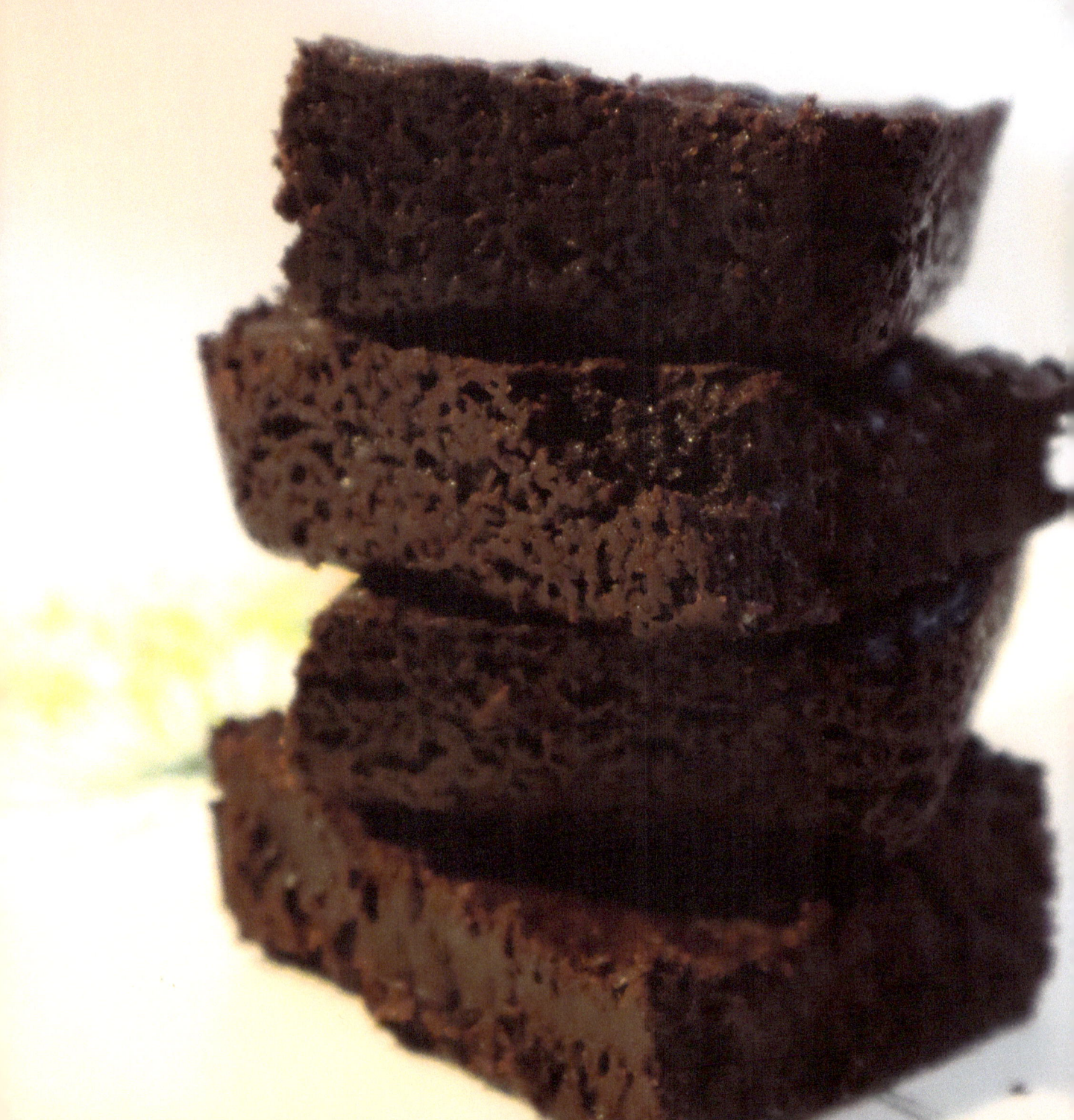

*Chocolate lovers, this one's for you. I took an already chocolatey brownie recipe and added **even more** chocolate. Fudgy brownies with so much chocolate they're simply decadent. Warm, wildly chocolatey brownies. RUN to your kitchen and make these delicious treats immediately.*

Serving:
12 brownies

Prep Time:
10 minutes

Bake Time:
30 minutes

Ingredients

- 1 stick (8 tbsp) softened butter
- ¾ cup semisweet chocolate chips
- ½ cup dark chocolate chips
- ¾ cup sugar
- 1 tbsp vanilla
- ½ tsp coffee granules
- 2 large eggs, room temp
- ¼ cup flour
- ⅓ cup cocoa powder
- ½ tsp baking powder

Directions

1. Preheat the oven to 350°F. Line a 9x9 or 8x8 inch pan with parchment paper.
2. Melt together butter, semisweet, and dark chocolate chips until smooth.
3. Stir in sugar, vanilla, and coffee.
4. In a separate bowl, whisk eggs for about a minute until slightly bubbly/foamy.
5. Mix eggs into chocolate mix.
6. Add flour, cocoa powder, and baking powder and mix until just combined.
7. Spread mixture into the baking pan.
8. Bake for 25-30 minutes or until just set.
9. Let cool for 5 minutes.
10. Enjoy!

Variations

- Swirl peanut butter through batter before baking.
- Mix raspberries through batter (may have to add a couple minutes to baking for extra moisture).
- Add extra chocolate chips and/or peanut butter chips into the batter before baking.
- Dust with powdered sugar or raspberry powder after baking.

Note:

Can use all semisweet or dark chocolate chips as preferred.

Coffee granules are optional—coffee just enhances chocolate flavor.

Cakes

Decadently Chocolate Brownies
continued

Double Recipe (24 brownies)

- 2 sticks (16 tbsp) softened butter
- 1 ½ cups semisweet chocolate chips
- 1 cup dark chocolate chips
- 1 ½ cups sugar
- 2 tbsp vanilla
- 1 tsp coffee granules
- 4 large eggs, room temp
- ½ cup flour
- ⅔ cup cocoa powder
- 1 tsp baking powder

(Use 2 pans)

Single Serve (4 brownies)

- ½ stick (4 tbsp) softened butter
- ¼ cup and 2 tbsp semisweet chocolate chips
- ¼ cup dark chocolate chips
- ¼ cup and 2 tbsp sugar
- ½ tbsp vanilla
- ¼ tsp coffee granules
- 1 large egg, room temp
- 2 tbsp cup flour
- 3 tbsp cocoa powder
- ¼ tsp baking powder

(Use smaller pan, reduce baking time to 15-20 minutes)

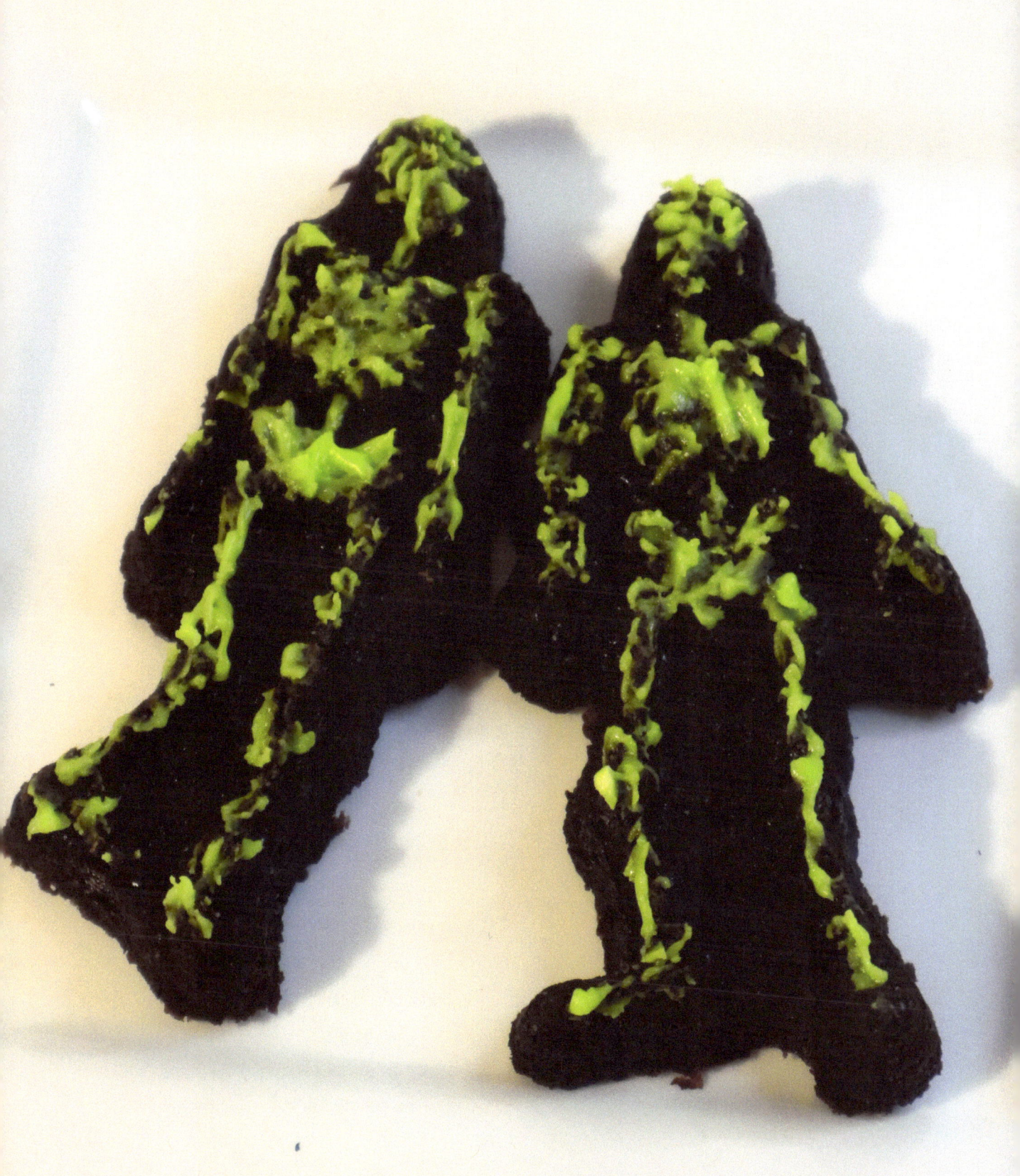

Mini Chocolate Peanut Butter Cheesecakes

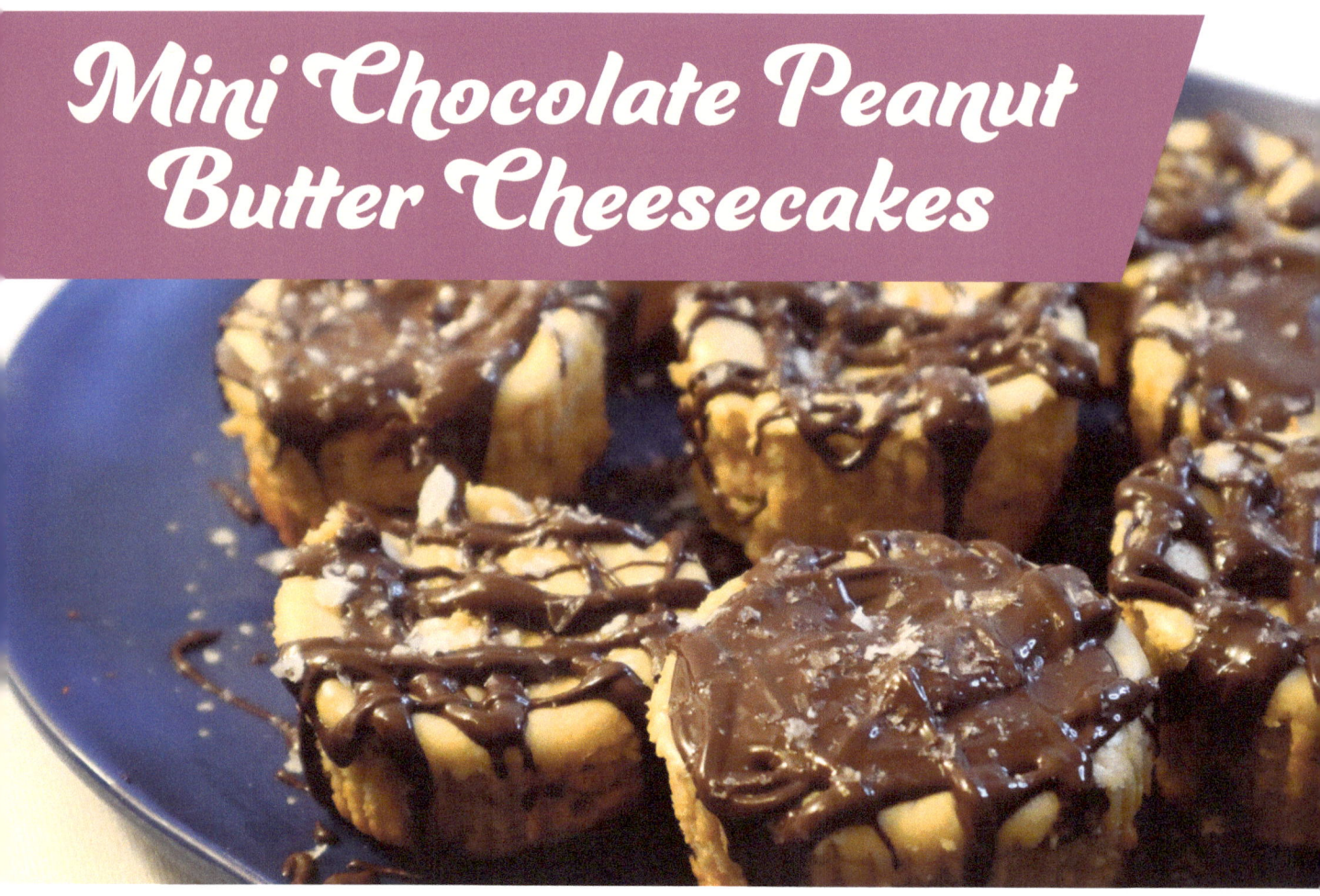

If there's a dessert combo I love more than chocolate and raspberries, it's chocolate and peanut butter. Perhaps the saying is "goes together like peanut butter and jelly" but seriously, it should really be "goes together like peanut butter and chocolate." Creamy peanut butter cheesecakes topped with homemade "magic shell" chocolate make for a very happy snack. Try one. Or two.

Serving:
24 cheesecakes

Prep Time:
10 minutes

Bake Time:
45 minutes

Ingredients

- 24 Oreos
- 2 packages cream cheese (16 oz)
- ⅔ cup sugar
- 2 eggs
- 2 tsp vanilla
- 1 cup vanilla yogurt
- ¾ cup creamy peanut butter
- 2 tbsp flour
- 1 cup semisweet chocolate chips
- 1 tsp coconut oil

Directions

1. Preheat the oven to 350°F. Line cupcake pan with paper liners and place an Oreo in the bottom each.
2. Beat cream cheese and peanut butter on medium speed until smooth.
3. Add sugar, eggs, vanilla and beat on medium speed until smooth.
4. Add yogurt and flour and beat on low speed until smooth.
5. Fill each cupcake liner about ⅔ full.
6. Bake for about 25 minutes until just barely set. Cool in the oven with the door cracked for 20 minutes.
7. While baking, heat chocolate chips and coconut oil until fully melted and stir until smooth.
8. Remove cheesecakes from the oven and place on the cooling rack.
9. Pour a thin layer of melted chocolate on each cheesecake and allow to cool and set.
10. Cover and place in the fridge until serving.
11. Enjoy!

Variations

- Use chunky peanut butter instead of creamy.
- Use peanut butter Oreos instead of regular.
- Use double stuff Oreos for crusts.
- Mix in 1 cup of diced apples.
- Dust with powdered sugar.
- Add sprinkles after adding chocolate coating but before chocolate sets.
- Replace peanut butter with pureed raspberries and/or other fruit of choice.

Double Recipe (48 cheesecakes)

- 48 Oreos
- 4 packages cream cheese (32 oz)
- 1⅓ cups sugar
- 4 eggs
- 4 tsp vanilla
- 2 cups vanilla yogurt
- 1½ cups creamy peanut butter
- ¼ cup flour
- 1½ cups semisweet chocolate chips
- 2 tsp coconut oil

Single Serve (12 cheesecakes)

- 12 Oreos
- 1 package cream cheese (8 oz)
- ⅓ cup sugar
- 1 eggs
- 1 tsp vanilla
- ½ cup vanilla yogurt
- ¼ cup and 2 tbsp creamy peanut butter
- 1 tbsp flour
- ½ cup semisweet chocolate chips
- ½ tsp coconut oil

Mom's Famous Chocolate Chip Cookies

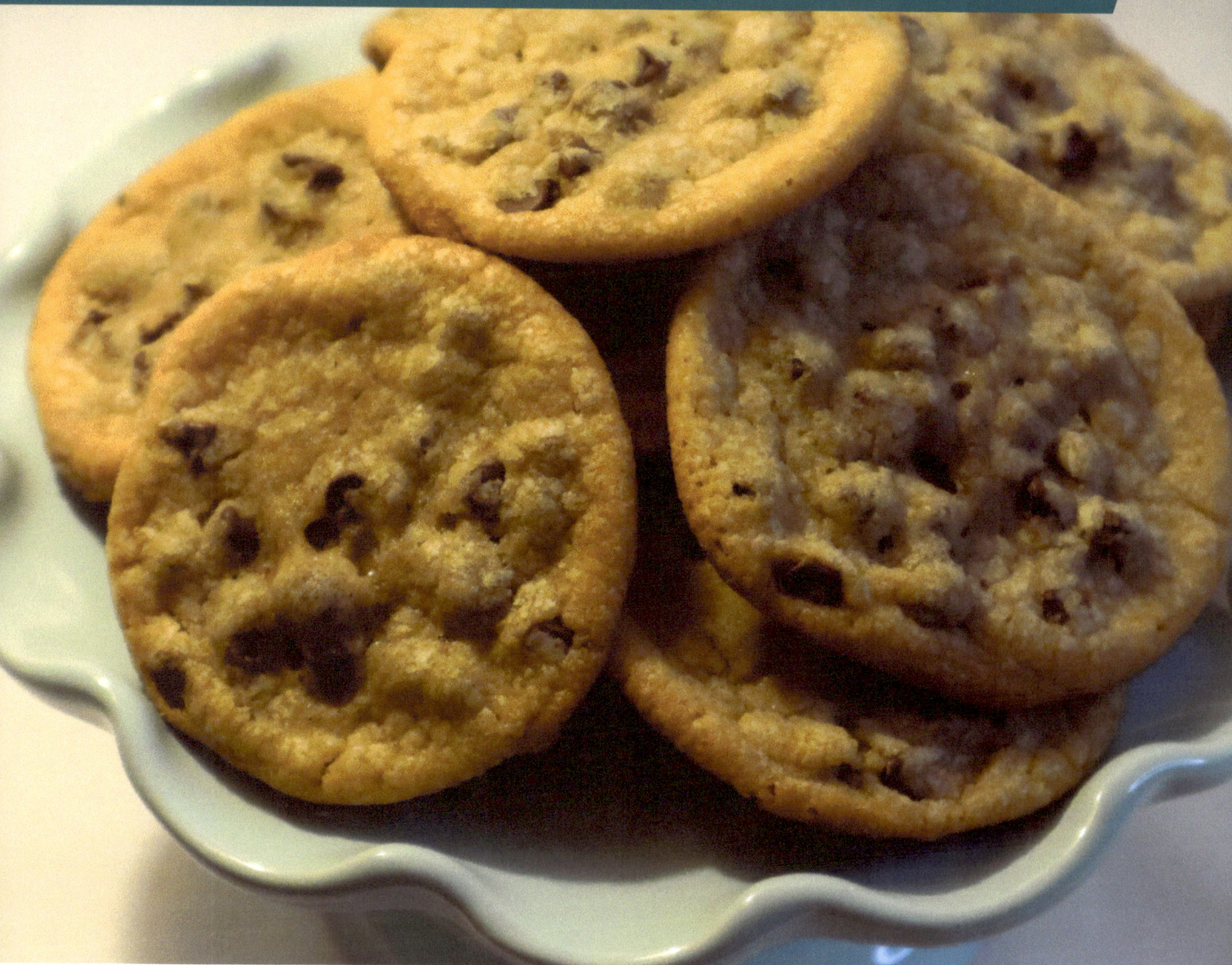

The recipe that started it all. I'm fairly certain this is the first recipe my mom taught me to bake. I have many, many fond childhood memories of these cookies (and my brothers and I swiping fingerfuls of the cookie dough when Mom wasn't looking. She was never fooled.) These cookies are soft, chewy mouthfuls of chocolate chip cookie perfection. Hot tip? After you've eaten your share warm from the oven, store them in your freezer. Take them out for a couple minutes before eating for bites of chewy bliss. Trust me.

Serving:
24 cookies

Prep Time:
15 minutes

Bake Time:
10 minutes

Ingredients

- ½ cup softened shortening
- ½ cup and 2 tbsp firmly packed brown sugar
- ½ cup and 2 tbsp granulated sugar
- ½ tsp vanilla
- ¼ tsp water
- 1 egg
- 1 cup flour
- ½ tsp baking soda
- ½ tsp salt
- ½ package chocolate chips

Directions

1. Preheat the oven to 350°F.
2. Beat shortening, sugars, vanilla, water, and eggs until light and fluffy.
3. Mix flour with salt and baking soda.
4. Blend into shortening mixture.
5. Stir in chips.
6. Drop by ½ tablespoonful onto an ungreased or parchment paper lined baking sheet.
7. Bake for 10 minutes.**

Note:
**These will look not quite done when you take them out—soft and puffy in the middle. DO NOT bake longer. You will be tempted but trust me and take them out. They will flatten as they cool and will be amazing and chewy!

Double Recipe (48 cookies)

- 1 cup softened shortening
- ¾ cup firmly packed brown sugar
- ¾ cup granulated sugar
- 1 tsp vanilla
- ½ tsp water
- 2 eggs
- 2 cups flour
- 1 tsp baking soda
- 1 tsp salt
- 1 package chocolate chips

Single Serve (12 cookies)

- ¼ cup softened shortening
- ¼ cup and 1 tbsp firmly packed brown sugar
- ¼ cup and 1 tbsp granulated sugar
- ¼ tsp vanilla
- ¼ tsp water
- ½ an egg
- ½ cup flour
- ¼ tsp baking soda
- ¼ tsp salt
- ¼ package chocolate chips

Chewy Chocolate Cookies

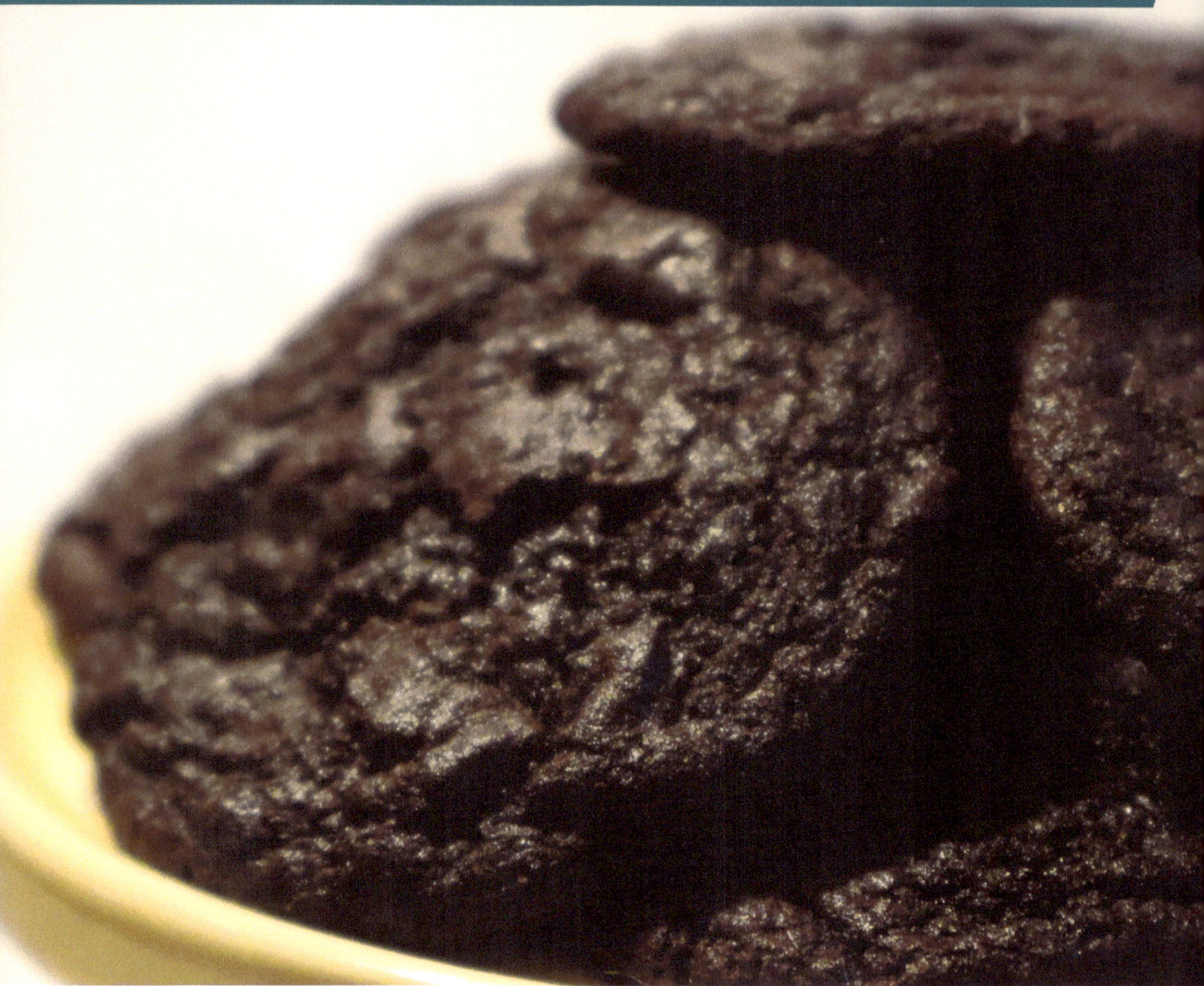

For years I thought of these as "Christmas cookies," which I'm aware is very different from most people's idea of Christmas cookies! For whatever reason, I only remember my mom making these mind-blowingly delicious cookies around Christmas and I was years out of college before it occurred to me I could make them any time of the year. (It took me a weirdly long time to realize that!) These soft, chewy cookies basically melt in your mouth and make your taste buds jump up and tango. Like my chocolate chip cookies, I like to store these in the freezer—even though they rarely last long enough to truly need freezing!

Serving:
~ 24 cookies

Prep Time:
10 minutes

Bake Time:
10 minutes

Ingredients

- 6 tbsp butter, softened
- 1 cup sugar
- 1 whole egg + 1 egg white
- 1 tsp vanilla
- 1 cup flour
- ½ cup and 2 tbsp cocoa powder
- ½ tsp baking soda
- ¼ tsp salt

Directions

1. Preheat the oven to 350°F.
2. Cream butter and sugar until light and fluffy.
3. Blend in egg, egg white and vanilla.
4. Combine flour, cocoa, baking soda, and salt.
5. Mix dry ingredients into a creamed mixture.
6. Drop teaspoons sized balls onto a parchment paper lined baking sheet.
7. Bake for 8-9 minutes—DO NOT OVERBAKE. They will look soft and puffy.** They will flatten as they cool.

Variations

- Dust with powdered sugar.
- Add peanut butter chips.
- Enclose 2-3 mini marshmallows in each ball of dough before baking.
- Sprinkle with flaky sea salt.
- Add mini M&Ms.

Note:
**These will look not quite done when you take them out—soft and puffy in the middle. DO NOT bake longer. You will be tempted but trust me and take them out. They will flatten as they cool and will be melt-in-your mouth amazing and chewy!

Double Recipe (54 cookies)

- 1 ¼ cups butter, softened
- 2 cups sugar
- 2 eggs + 1 egg white
- 2 tsp vanilla
- 2 cups flour
- ¾ cup cocoa powder
- 1 tsp baking soda
- ½ tsp salt

Single Serve (12 cookies)

- 3 tbsp butter, softened
- ½ cup sugar
- 1 egg
- ½ tsp vanilla
- ½ cup flour
- ¼ cup and 1 tbsp cocoa powder
- ¼ tsp baking soda
- ⅛ tsp salt

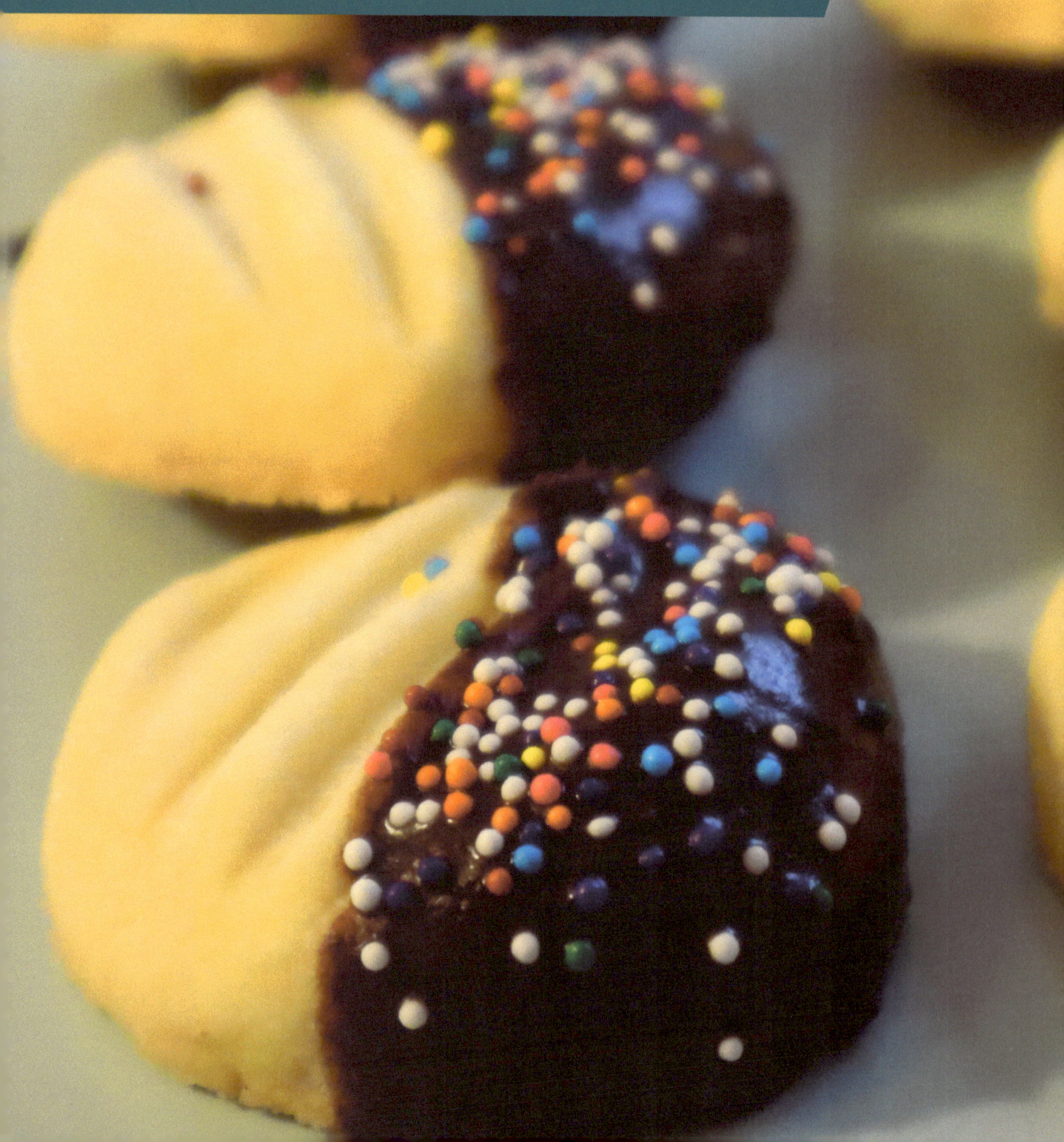
Whipped Shortbread Cookies

These are not your typical crumbly shortbread. These are soft, melt-in-your mouth wonders of EAT ME NOW. Simple, quick, and damn right delicious.

Serving:
12 cookies

Prep Time:
10 minutes

Bake Time:
20 minutes

Ingredients

- 6 tbsp butter, softened
- 3 tbsp powdered sugar
- ½ cup and 1 tbsp flour
- 3 tbsp cornstarch

Directions

1. Beat butter and powdered sugar until light and fluffy (about 3-4 minutes).
2. Beat in flour and cornstarch just until combined.
3. Roll into 12 cookie balls, then press tops with a cookie press or fork.
4. Set the baking sheet in the freezer for 10-15 minutes while the oven preheats to 300°F.
5. Bake for about 20 minutes until the tops look just set and very lightly brown on edges.
6. Enjoy!

Variations

- Add chocolate chips to cookie dough.
- Add peanut butter (about ¼ cup) to cookie dough.
- Top with sprinkles prior to baking.
- Mix raspberry/strawberry powder into cookie dough.
- Dip half cookie in melted chocolate after baking.
- Drizzle finished cookies with melted chocolate.

Double Recipe (24 cookies)

- 12 tbsp butter, softened
- 6 tbsp powdered sugar
- 1 cup and 2 tbsp flour
- 6 tbsp cornstarch

Single Serve (6 cookies)

- 3 tbsp butter, softened
- 1 ½ tbsp powdered sugar
- ¼ cup and ½ tbsp flour
- 1 ½ tbsp cornstarch

Homemade Oreos

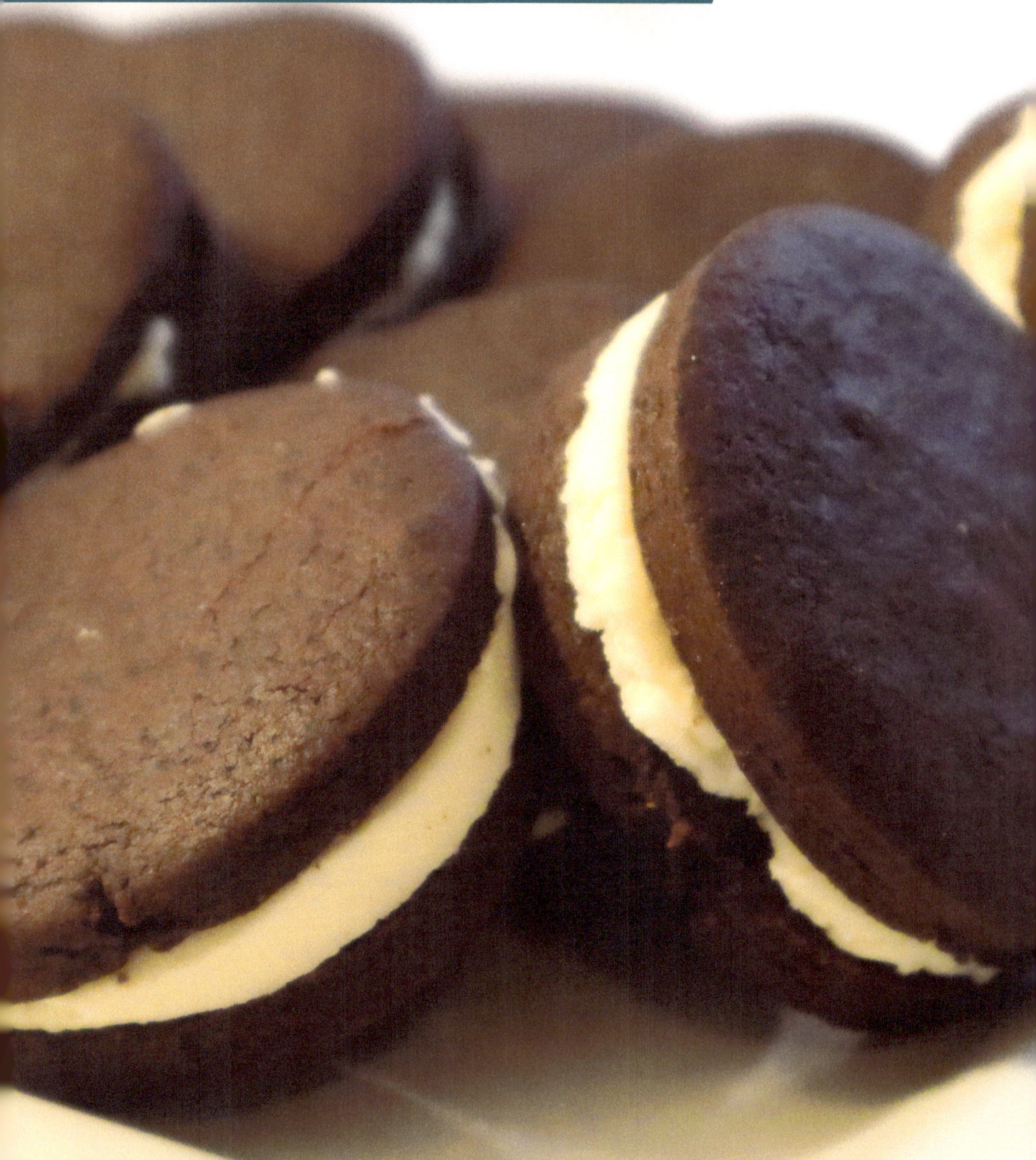

Anyone remember brownie Oreos? Do they still make those? These are a kind of hybrid between regular Oreos and brownie Oreos, making the absolute best of both worlds. Honestly, though, I could just eat the cream filling by itself. It tastes just like the real deal.

Serving:
10 cookies

Prep Time:
1 hour

Bake Time:
8-10 minutes

Ingredients

Cookies

- ¾ cup sugar
- 1 cup butter, room temp (2 sticks)
- 1 tsp baking powder
- 1 tsp vanilla
- ½ tsp espresso powder
- ¾ tsp salt
- 1 large egg
- ½ cup cocoa powder
- 2 ¼ cups flour

Filling

- 4 tbsp butter, softened
- 4 tbsp shortening, room temp
- 1 ¾ cups powdered sugar
- 1 tsp vanilla

Directions

Cookies

1. Beat together the sugar, butter, baking powder, vanilla, espresso powder, and salt until fluffy. Scrape sides and bottom of bowl.
2. Beat in egg and scrape bowl again.
3. Whisk together flour and cocoa, then add to egg and butter mixture until well blended.
4. Refrigerate for 30 minutes.
5. Preheat the oven to 375°F. Lightly grease 2 baking sheets.
6. Divide dough in half. Sprinkle with extra cocoa to keep from sticking.
7. Roll dough to ¼ to ⅛ inch thickness.
8. Cut into desired shapes with a cookie cutter. Place on baking sheets.
9. Bake for 8-10 minutes until the edges are firm.
10. Remove from the oven and allow them to cool completely.

Filling

11. Beat butter and shortening together until creamy and combined.
12. Add powdered sugar and vanilla, beat on low for 1 minute and then high for 1 minute until creamy and combined. The filling will be thick.
13. Spread filling between two cooled cookies. Repeat until all are filled.
14. Enjoy!

Homemade Oreos

continued

Variations

- Add tbsp peanut butter to filling for Peanut Butter Oreos.
- Add mint extract, peppermint extract, etc. for different flavored fillings.

Double Recipe (20 cookies)

Cookies

- 1 ½ cups sugar
- 2 cups butter, room temp (4 sticks)
- 2 tsp baking powder
- 2 tsp vanilla
- 1 tsp espresso powder
- 1 ½ tsp salt
- 2 large eggs
- 1 cup cocoa powder
- 4 ½ cups flour

Filling

- 4 tbsp butter, softened
- 4 tbsp vegetable shortening, room temp
- 1 ¾ cups powdered sugar
- 1 tsp vanilla

Single Serve (5 cookies)

Cookies

- ¼ cup + 2 tbsp sugar
- ½ cup butter, room temp (1 stick)
- ½ tsp baking powder
- ½ tsp vanilla
- ¼ tsp espresso powder
- ¼ tsp salt
- ½ large egg
- ¼ cup cocoa powder
- 1 cup + 2 tbsp flour

Filling

- 1 tbsp butter, softened
- 1 tbsp vegetable shortening, room temp
- ½ cup powdered sugar
- ¼ tsp vanilla

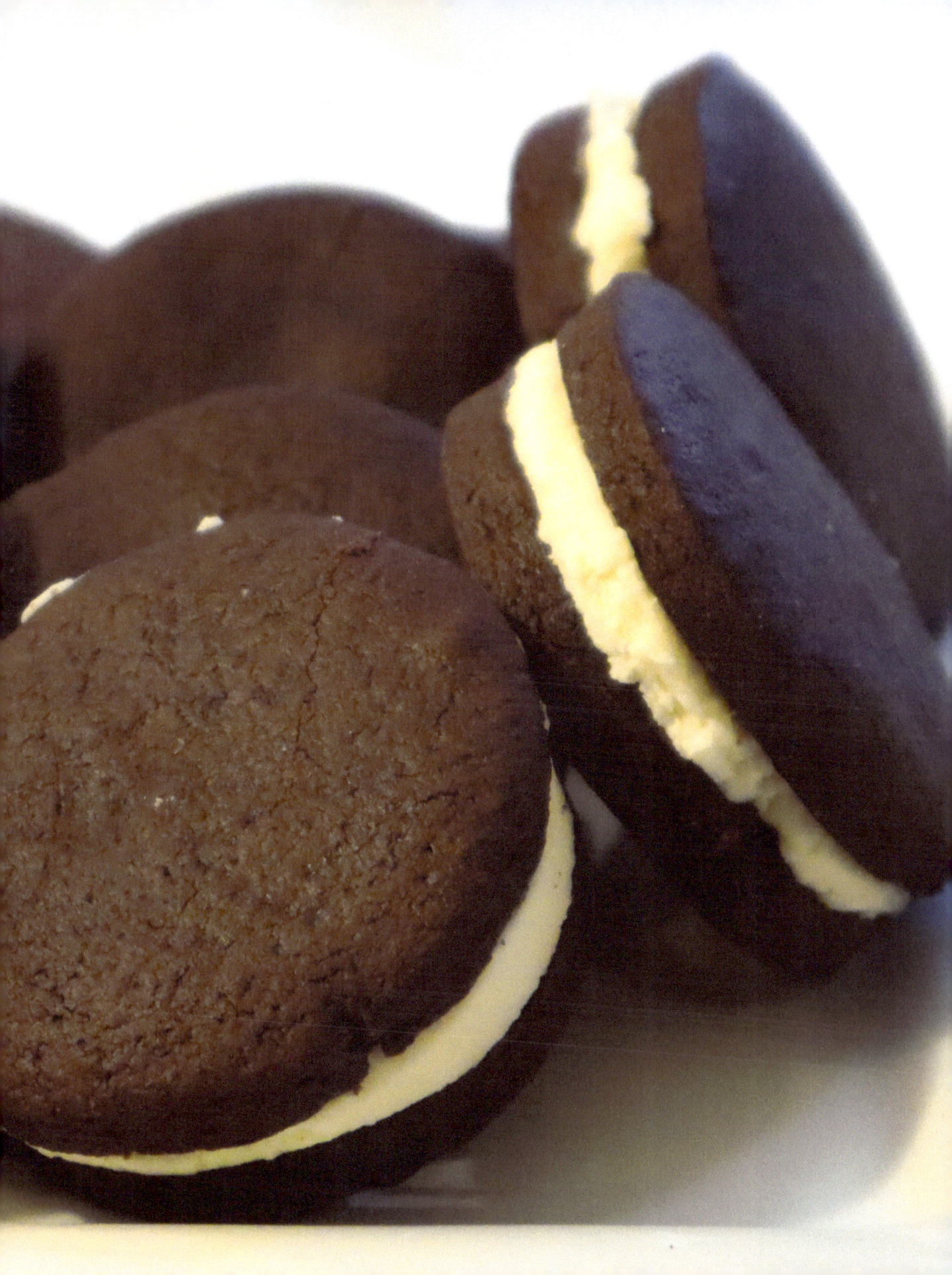

Sugar Cookies

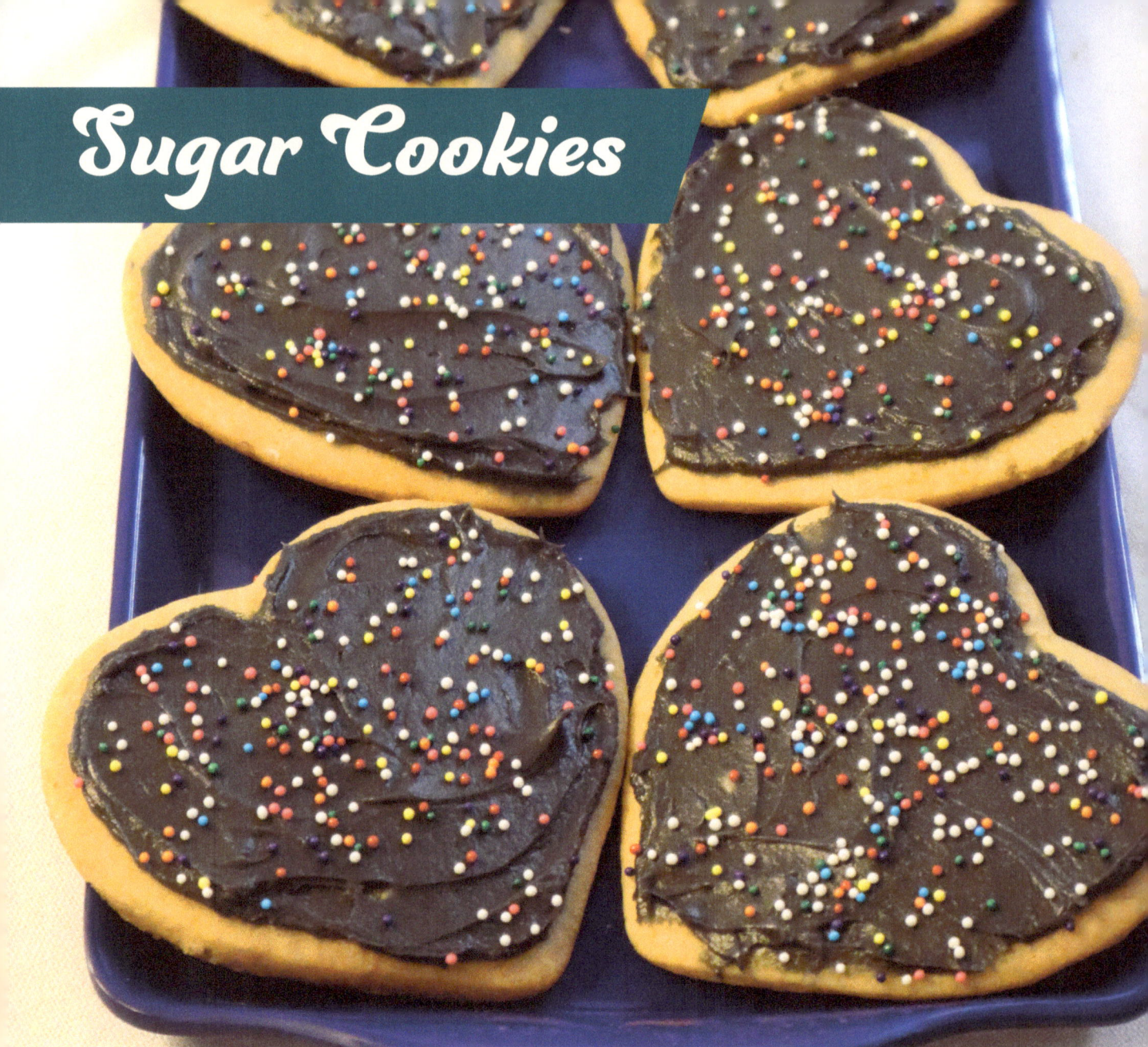

I don't remember making sugar cookies much as a kid, we were very much a chocolate chip cookie family. So, for a long time, I wasn't much of a sugar cookie fan—store bought ones always tasted kind of stale and hard to me. Then I was introduced to homemade sugar cookies that were soft, fresh, and delicious. Chocolate chip may always be my first love, but I probably won't turn down a good homemade sugar cookie!

Serving:
22 cookies

Prep Time:
20 minutes

Bake Time:
15 minutes

Ingredients

- ¾ cup butter, room temp (1 ½ sticks)
- ¾ cup packed brown sugar
- 2 tsp vanilla
- 1 egg, room temp
- 2 cups flour
- ½ tsp baking soda
- ½ tsp salt

Directions

1. Cream together the butter and brown sugar until light and fluffy.
2. Add vanilla and egg, mix until combined.
3. Add flour, baking soda, and salt, beat until combined and starts to form a rough ball.
4. Roll out half the dough on a floured surface to about ¼ in thickness. Cut out with your preferred cookie cutter.
5. Transfer carefully to a parchment lined baking sheet.
6. Preheat the oven to 350°F. In the meantime, place cutout cookies into the freezer for 10-20 minutes. (This will help them hold their shape.)
7. Bake cookies for 8-10 minutes, or until just lightly golden. Cool on a baking sheet for 5 minutes and transfer to the cooling rack.
8. Frost with choice of frosting (royal, cream cheese, buttercream, etc.) *See recipes in Frostings & Fillings.*

Variations

- Add cinnamon or extracts for added flavors.

Double Recipe (44 cookies)

- 1 ½ cups butter, room temp (3 sticks)
- 1 ½ cups packed brown sugar
- 4 tsp vanilla
- 2 eggs, room temp
- 4 cups flour
- 1 tsp baking soda
- 1 tsp salt

Single Serve (10 cookies)

- 6 tbsp butter, room temp
- ¼ cup + 2 tbsp packed brown sugar
- 1 tsp vanilla
- ½ egg, room temp
- 1 cup flour
- ¼ tsp baking soda
- ¼ tsp salt

Smash Cookies

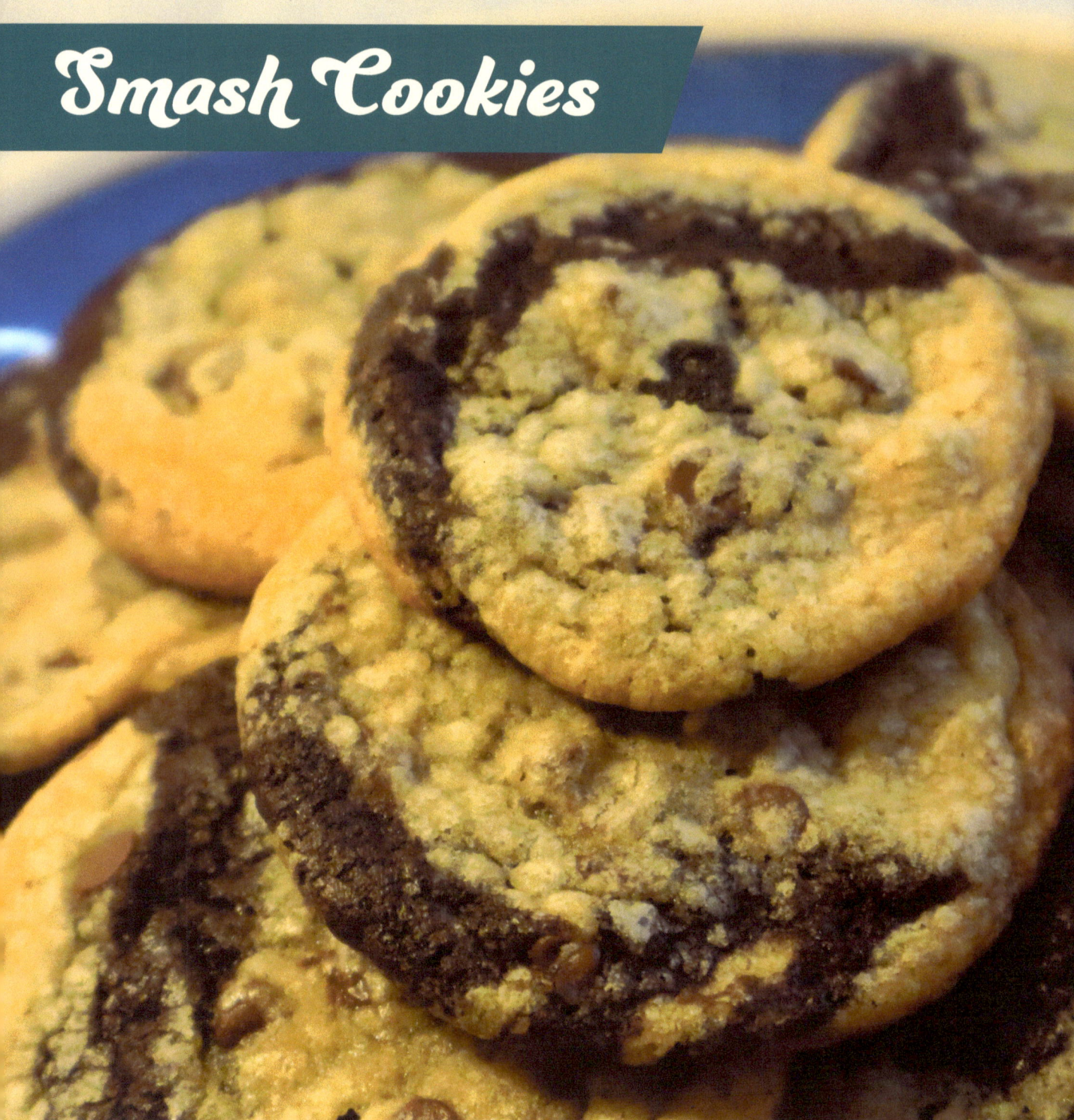

Ah, smash cookies. So named because I basically smashed together my two favorite cookie recipes into one round swirl of delectable goodness. Chocolate chip cookie swirled with chewy chocolate cookie for the best of both worlds brought together. Smash together, friends, and taste the joy.

Serving:
24 cookies

Prep Time:
20 minutes

Bake Time:
20 minutes

Ingredients

Chocolate Chip Cookie Dough

- ½ cup softened shortening
- ½ cup + 2 tbsp firmly packed brown sugar
- ½ cup + 2 tbsp granulated sugar
- ½ tsp vanilla
- ¼ tsp water
- 1 egg
- 1 cup flour
- ½ tsp baking soda
- ½ tsp salt
- ½ package chocolate chips

Chocolate Cookie Dough

- 3 tbsp softened butter
- ½ cup sugar
- 1 egg
- ½ tsp vanilla
- ½ cup flour
- ¼ cup + 1 tbsp cocoa powder
- ¼ tsp baking soda
- ⅛ tsp salt

Directions

Chocolate Chip Cookie Dough

1. Preheat the oven to 350°F.
2. Beat shortening, sugars, vanilla, water, and eggs until light and fluffy.
3. Mix flour with salt and baking soda.
4. Blend into shortening mixture.
5. Stir in chips.
6. Set aside while making chocolate cookie dough.

Chocolate Cookie Dough

7. Cream butter and sugar until light and fluffy.
8. Blend in egg, egg white and vanilla.
9. Combine flour, cocoa, baking soda, and salt.
10. Mix dry ingredients into the creamed mixture.

Combine

11. Roll out chocolate chip cookie dough between two sheets of parchment paper sprayed with cooking oil to about ¼ of an inch thick.
12. Remove top parchment paper sheet and spread chocolate cookie dough over chocolate chip dough. (This will be messy and does not need to be perfect!)
13. Using bottom parchment paper, fold ⅓ dough over onto itself. Then repeat with the opposite ⅓ of the dough. This creates layers.
14. Cut folded dough into roughly 1-inch by 1-inch squares and roll into balls.
15. Place balls a few inches apart on a baking sheet.
16. Bake for 9-10 minutes until slightly browned on edges but soft and puffy in the middle. (They will not look quite done but take them out anyway!) They will flatten as they cool and be wonderfully chewy!

Smash Cookies
continued

Double Recipe (48 cookies)

Chocolate Chip Dough
- 1 cup softened shortening
- 1 ¼ cups firmly packed brown sugar
- 1 ¼ cups granulated sugar
- 1 tsp vanilla
- ½ tsp water
- 2 eggs
- 2 cups flour
- 1 tsp baking soda
- 1 tsp salt
- 1 package chocolate chips

Chocolate Cookie Dough
- 6 tbsp softened butter
- 1 cup sugar
- 2 whole eggs + 1 egg white
- 1 tsp vanilla
- 1 cup flour
- ¾ cocoa powder
- ½ tsp baking soda
- ¼ tsp salt

Single Serve (12 cookies)

Chocolate Chip Dough
- ¼ cup softened shortening
- ¼ cup + 1 tbsp firmly packed brown sugar
- ¼ cup + 1 tbsp granulated sugar
- ¼ tsp vanilla
- ⅛ tsp water
- ½ egg
- ½ cup flour
- ¼ tsp baking soda
- ¼ tsp salt
- ¼ package chocolate chips

Chocolate Cookie Dough
- 1 ½ tbsp softened butter
- ¼ cup sugar
- 1 whole egg
- ¼ tsp vanilla
- ¼ cup flour
- 3 ½ tbsp cocoa powder
- ⅛ tsp baking soda
- Pinch of salt

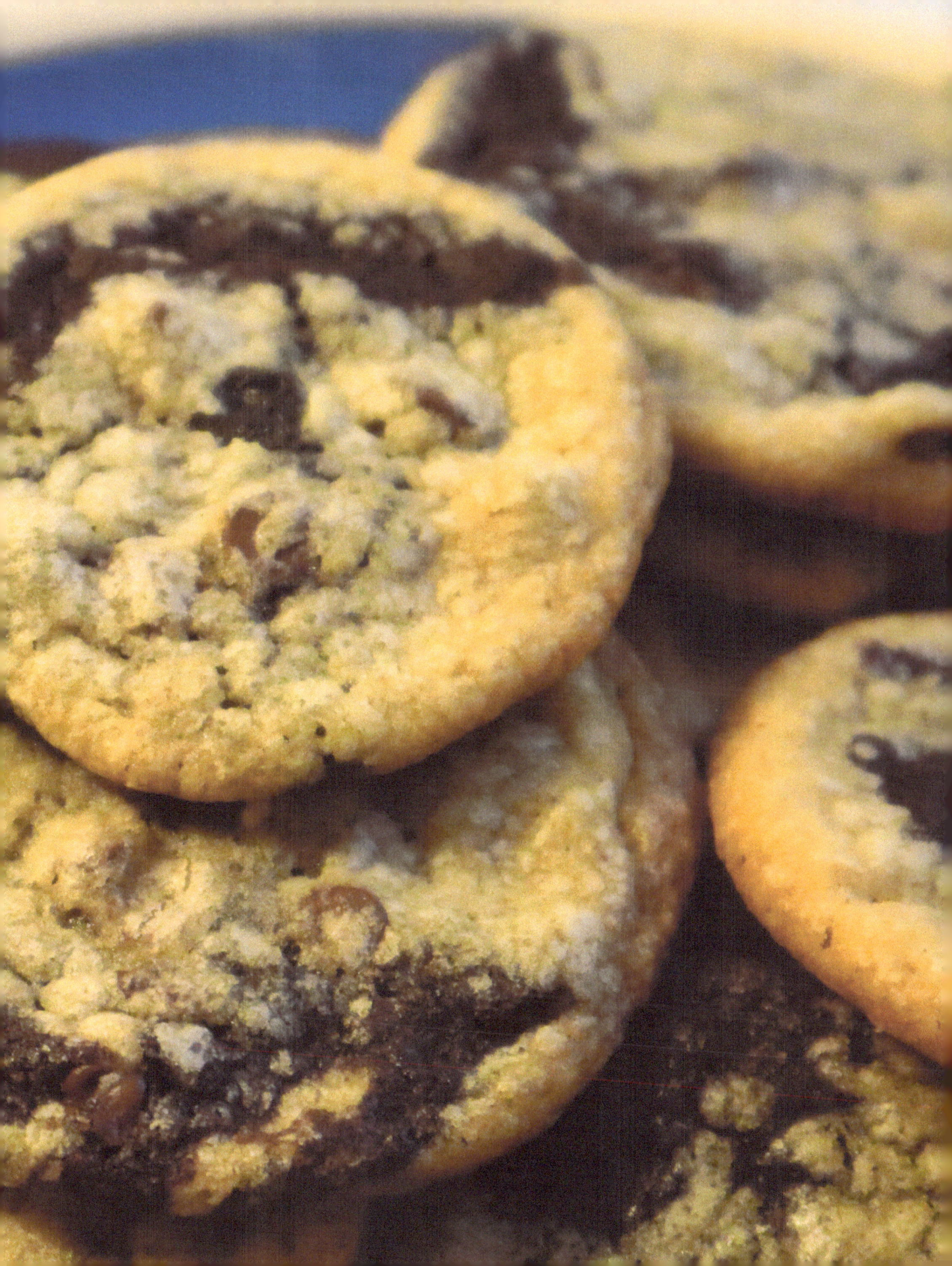

Raspberry Sugar Cookies

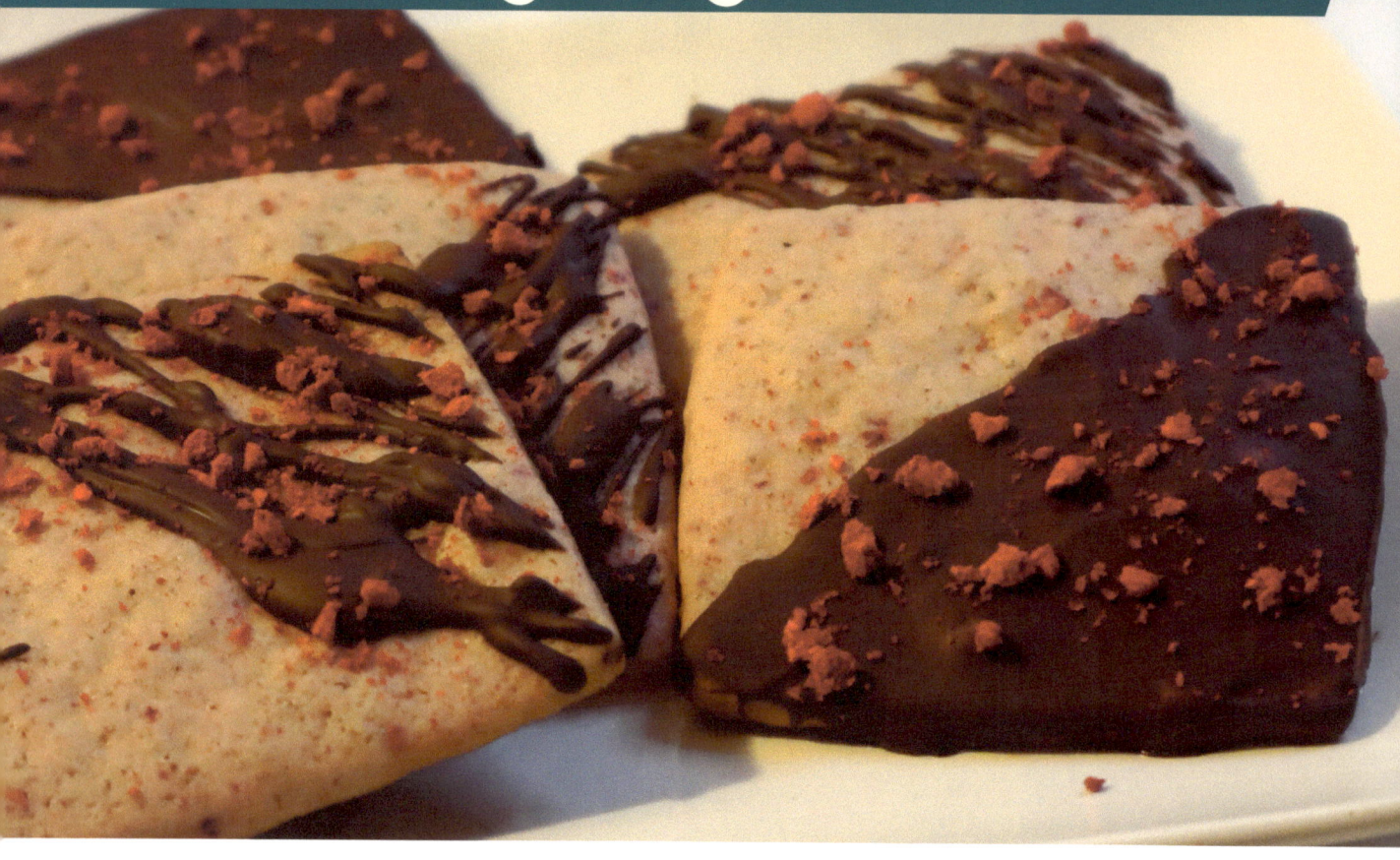

This recipe was inspired by the same little girl who inspired the Raspberry Lemonade later in the book. Sonya requested a "square cookie with chocolate chips." These are what was born from that request. And I do highly recommend adding mini chocolate chips to this cookie dough!

Serving:
12 cookies

Prep Time:
40 minutes

Bake Time:
10-15 minutes

Ingredients

- ½ bag of freeze dried raspberries
- ¾ cup flour
- ½ tsp baking powder
- ¼ tsp salt
- 4 tbsp softened butter (unsalted)
- ¼ cup sugar
- ½ egg
- ½ tsp vanilla
- ¼ tsp almond extract

Directions

1. Make raspberry powder. Process freeze dried raspberries in a food processor until they become a fine powder. Sift through a fine strainer to remove any seeds.
2. Whisk together flour, baking powder, and salt. Set aside.
3. In a separate bowl, beat butter and sugar until light and fluffy.
4. Add egg, vanilla, almond extract, and 3 teaspoons raspberry powder.
5. Beat until well combined. Blend in flour mixture.
6. Roll out dough between two sheets of parchment paper until about ¼ inch thick (⅛ inch for slightly crispier cookies).
7. Chill dough for about 15 minutes in refrigerator.
8. Cut out cookies with desired cookie cutters.
9. While the oven preheats to 350°F, put cookies on a cookie sheet (don't overcrowd) in the freezer for 10-15 minutes.
10. If topping with sprinkles or coarse sugar, do so before baking.
11. Bake 8-12 minutes or until bottom edges are beginning to lightly brown.
12. Cool on a cooling rack.
13. Frost or decorate as desired.

Variations

- Dust with extra raspberry powder for added raspberry zip.
- Add mini chocolate chips to cookie batter.
- Dip half cookie in melted chocolate and dust with raspberry powder.
- Substitute strawberry powder for raspberry.
- Decorate with frosting of choice.

Note: Store leftover raspberry powder for future recipes

Double Recipe (24 cookies)

- 1 bag of freeze dried raspberries
- 1 ½ cups flour
- 1 tsp baking powder
- ½ tsp salt
- 8 tbsp softened butter (unsalted)
- ½ cup sugar
- 1 egg
- 1 tsp vanilla
- ¼ tsp almond extract

Single Serve (6 cookies)

- ¼ bag of freeze dried raspberries
- ¼ cup and 2 tbsp flour
- ¼ tsp baking powder
- ⅛ tsp salt
- 2 tbsp softened butter (unsalted)
- 2 tbsp sugar
- ¼ egg
- ¼ tsp vanilla
- ⅛ tsp almond extract

Strawberry Cheesecake Stuffed Cookies

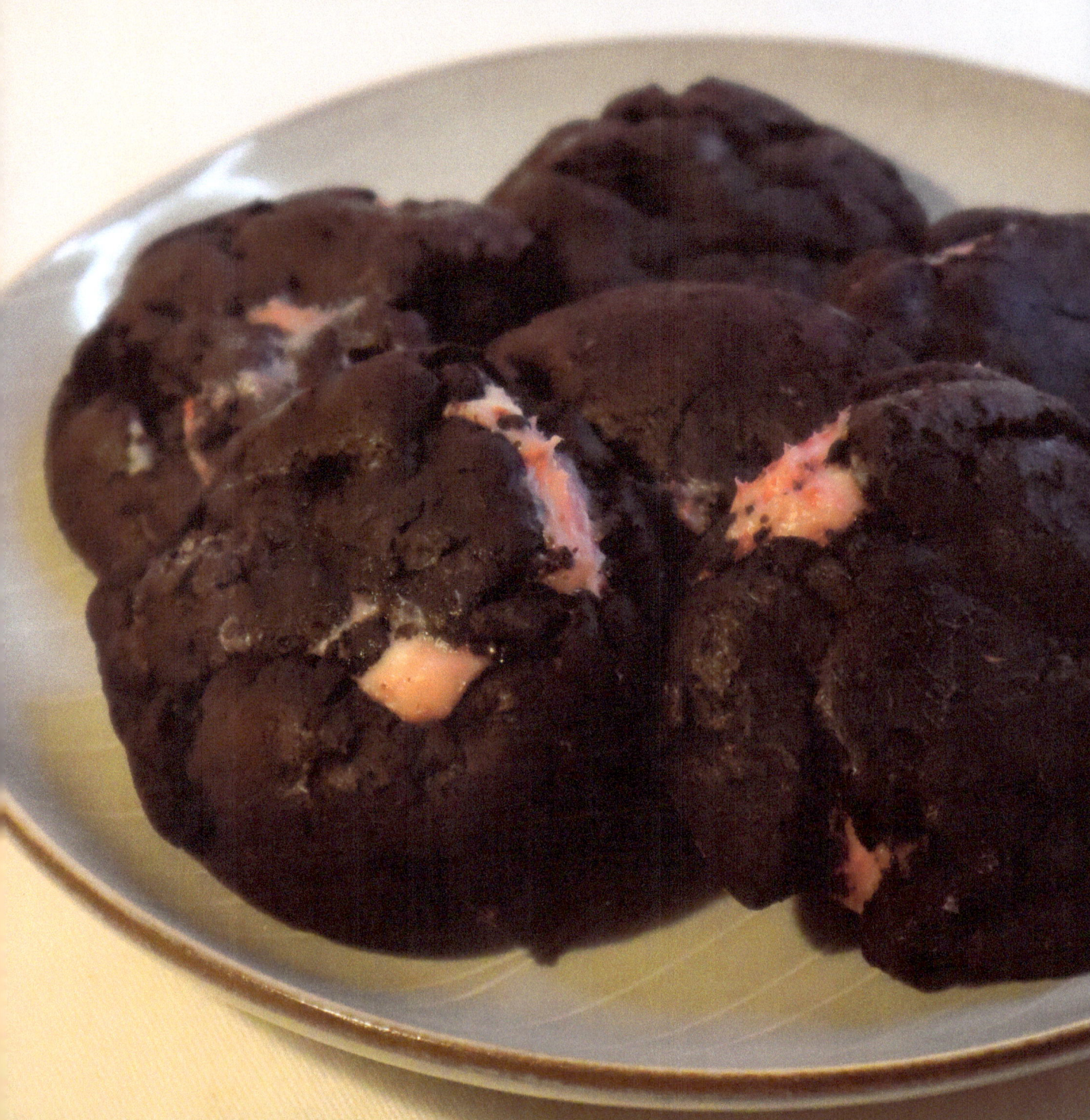

One of my favorite things is to experiment with what I can stuff into the Chewy Chocolate Cookie dough. Strawberry cream cheese has become a fast favorite! Sweet, slightly tangy cream cheese encased in chewy chocolate cookie dough is a symphony of yum, nom, and Mmmmm.

Serving:
12 cookies

Prep Time:
20 minutes

Bake Time:
20 minutes

Ingredients

- 6 tbsp softened butter
- 1 cup sugar
- 1 whole egg + 1 egg white
- 1 tsp vanilla
- 1 cup flour
- ½ cup + 2 tbsp cocoa powder
- ½ tsp baking soda
- ¼ tsp salt

Cream Cheese Filling

- 2 blocks cream cheese (16 oz)
- 4 tbsp freeze-dried strawberry powder
- ⅓ cup powdered sugar

Directions

1. Preheat the oven to 350°F.
2. Cream butter and sugar until light and fluffy.
3. Blend in egg, egg white and vanilla.
4. Combine flour, cocoa, baking soda, and salt.
5. Mix dry ingredients into a creamed mixture.
6. In another bowl, whip cream cheese with strawberry powder and powdered sugar until well combined.
7. Divide cream cheese into approximately 1 – 1 ½ tbsp sized balls.
8. Enclose each cream cheese ball with chocolate dough until covered.
9. Drop onto a parchment paper lined baking sheet.
10. Bake for 8-9 minutes—DO NOT OVERBAKE. They will look soft and puffy.** They will flatten as they cool.

Variations

- Substitute other freeze dried fruit powders.
- Use plain cream cheese.
- Use cinnamon instead of fruit flavoring.

Note:

**These will look not quite done when you take them out—soft and puffy in the middle. DO NOT bake longer. You will be tempted but trust me and take them out. They will flatten as they cool and will be melt-in-your mouth amazing and chewy!

Strawberry Cheesecake Stuffed Cookies

continued

Double Recipe (24 cookies)

- 1 ¼ cups softened butter
- 2 cups sugar
- 2 eggs + 1 egg white
- 2 tsp vanilla
- 2 cups flour
- ¾ cup cocoa powder
- 1 tsp baking soda
- ½ tsp salt

Cream Cheese Filling

- 4 blocks cream cheese (32 oz)
- 8 tbsp freeze-dried strawberry powder
- ⅔ cup powdered sugar

Single Serve (6 cookies)

- 3 tbsp softened butter
- ½ cup sugar
- 1 egg
- ½ tsp vanilla
- ½ cup flour
- ¼ cup + 1 tbsp cocoa powder
- ¼ tsp baking soda
- ⅛ tsp salt

Cream Cheese Filling

- 1 blocks cream cheese (8 oz)
- 2 tbsp freeze-dried strawberry powder
- 3 tbsp powdered sugar

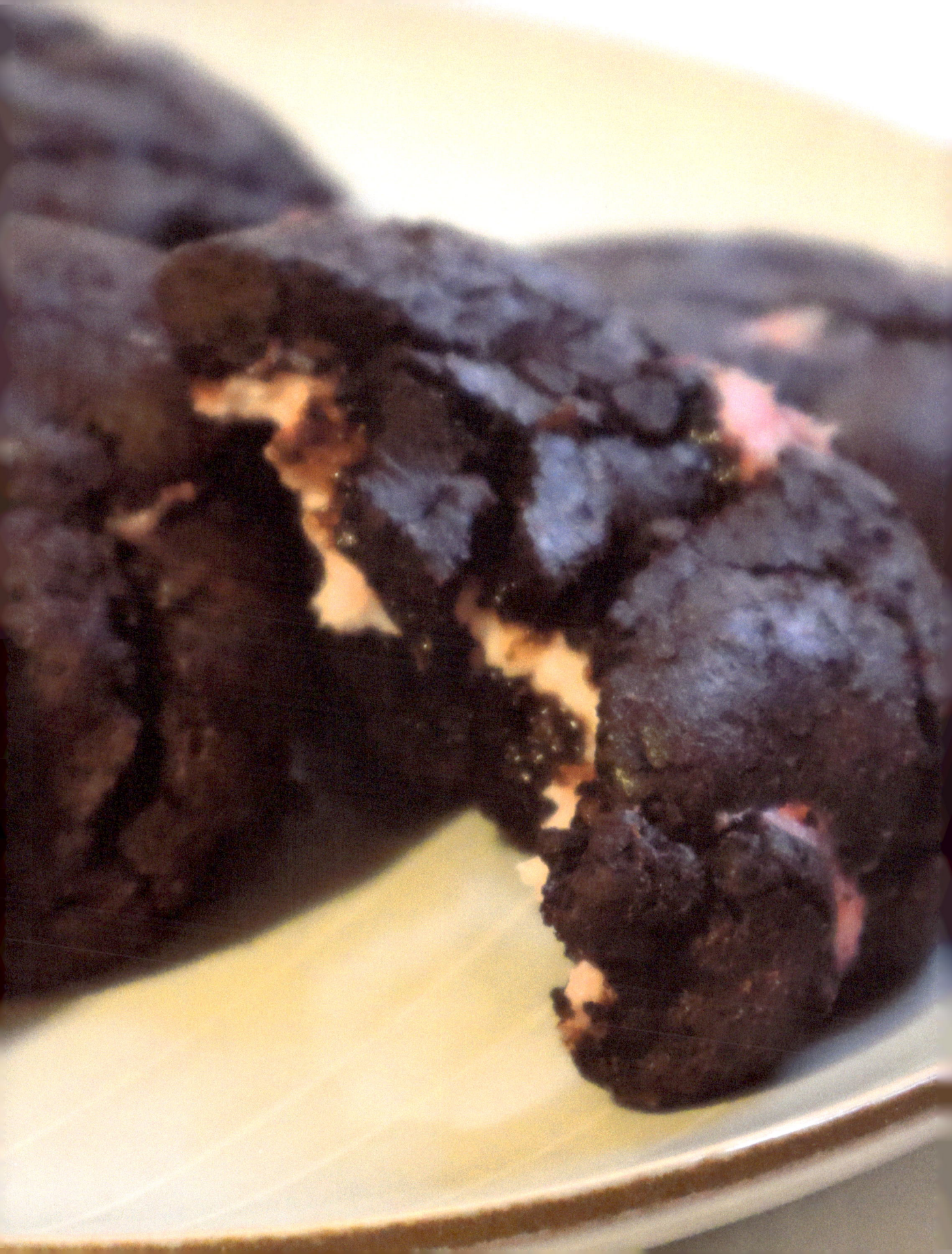

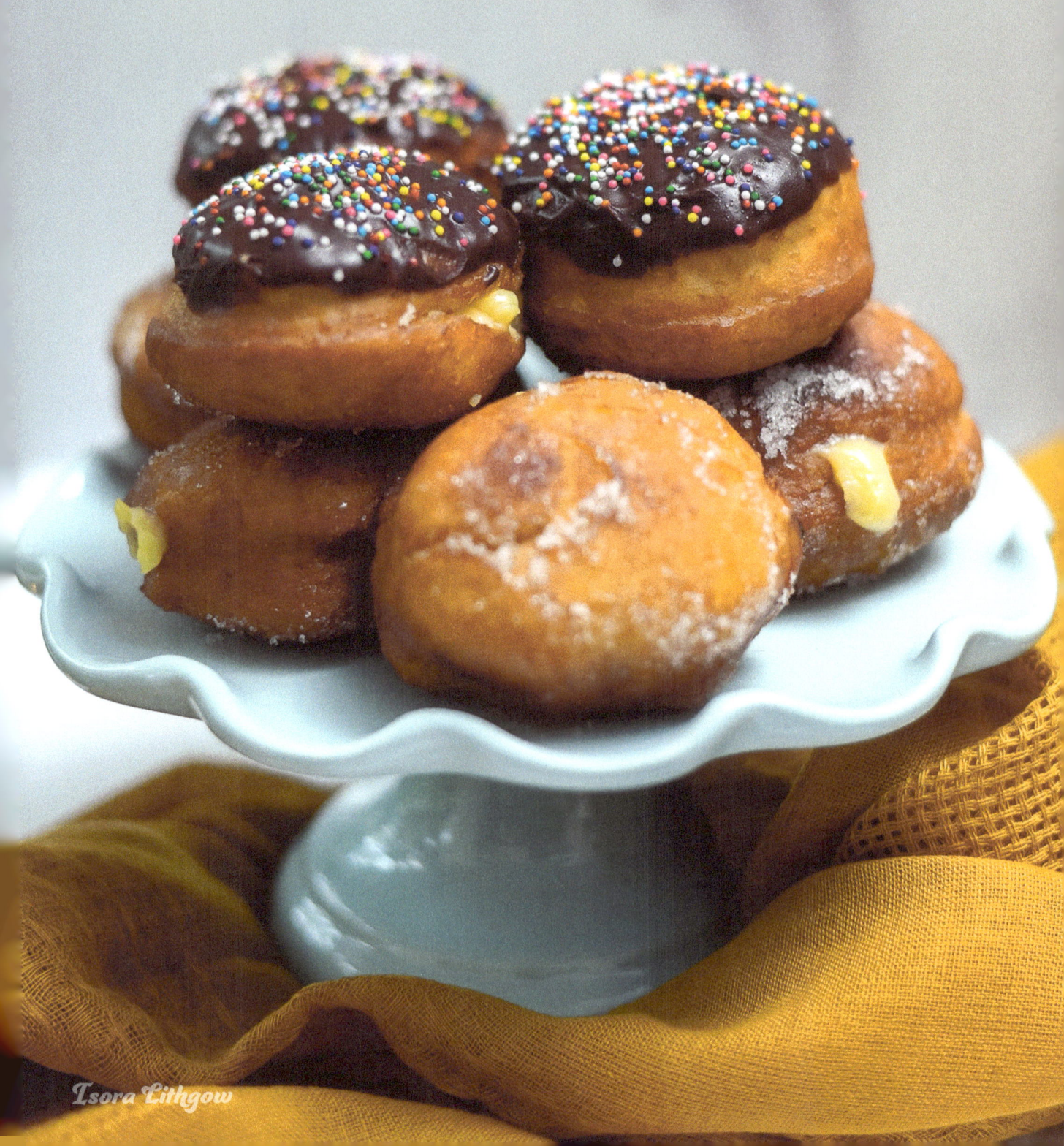

Cream Filled Beignets

I'm generally not a big donut person, but once again Mirabelles in Burlington VT's deliciousness inspired me. Their beignets make a regular appearance in my belly and I got curious about how to make them. This recipe is the tasty result! Have fun with different fillings and toppings and use your preference of air fryer or hot oil for baking!

Serving:
9 beignets

Prep Time:
2 hours

Bake Time:
5 minutes

Just for Fun Treats

Ingredients

Dough

- 1 ½ cups flour
- ½ cup milk
- 1 tbsp butter
- 1 tbsp brown sugar
- 1 + ⅛ tsp instant yeast
- 1 medium egg
- ¾ tsp salt
- ½ tsp vanilla

Pastry Cream

- 1 cup milk
- ½ tsp vanilla
- ⅛ tsp cornstarch
- 2 tbsp + 2 tsp sugar
- 2 egg yolk
- Optional: powdered sugar, chocolate ganache

Directions

Dough

1. Mix flour, salt, and yeast.
2. Heat milk until boiling hot.
3. In a separate bowl, combine butter and sugar and pour hot milk over top. Stir until butter is melted and sugar dissolved.
4. Allow to cool to lukewarm temp.
5. Add egg and vanilla and mix thoroughly.
6. Add wet ingredients to dry and mix until dough is formed. Knead for 3-5 minutes.
7. Place in a lightly oiled bowl and cover for about an hour or until doubled in size.
8. Roll dough out to about ¼ inch thick on a floured surface and cut into squares or circles. (I often use a large biscuit cutter.)
9. Set dough aside for 30 minutes or until doubled in size. While dough is resting, make pastry cream.

Pastry Cream

10. Combine ¾ cup milk and vanilla in a medium saucepan. Cook over high heat until just beginning to simmer, stirring often. Remove from heat.
11. In a medium bowl, whisk remaining milk, egg yolk, sugar, and cornstarch.

Cream Filled Beignets

continued

12. While whisking vigorously, slowly pour hot milk into the egg mixture.
13. Return mixture to saucepan and cook over high heat, continuously whisking until it thickens and begins to boil.
14. Pass through a strainer and into a bowl.
15. Place plastic wrap directly on top of pastry cream to prevent a skin from forming.
16. Cool to room temperature, then place in the fridge for 2-3 hours to set. Whip before use.//
17. **Air fryer:** Set to 390°F and cook for 3-5 minutes,** flipping halfway through. Brush with melted butter after removing.

    Oil: Pour several inches of oil in a large pan or fryer. Drop in and cook until golden brown. Remove and drain.
18. When cool enough to handle, cut a small slit and carefully create a pocket in beignet.
19. Fill the pastry bag with pastry cream and carefully fill each beignet with cream.
20. Top with powdered sugar or chocolate ganache or roll in sugar as desired.

Variations

- Use a variety of flavors for pastry cream—chocolate, vanilla, raspberry, lime, lemon, etc.
- Substitute pastry cream for jam or pudding.

Note:

**Air Fryer temps can vary, watch the first couple carefully to determine proper timing and temperature.

Double Recipe (18 beignets)

Dough
- 3 cups flour
- 1 cup milk
- 2 tbsp butter
- 2 tbsp brown sugar
- 2 ¼ tsp instant yeast
- 2 medium eggs
- 1 ½ tsp salt
- 1 tsp vanilla

Pastry Cream
- 2 cups milk
- 1 tsp vanilla
- ¼ tsp cornstarch
- ¼ cup + 1 tbsp sugar
- 4 egg yolk
- Optional: powdered sugar, chocolate ganache

Single Serve (4-5 beignets)

Dough
- ¾ cups flour
- ¼ cup milk
- ½ tbsp butter
- ½ tbsp brown sugar
- ½ tsp instant yeast
- ½ medium egg
- ¼ tsp + pinch of salt
- ¼ tsp vanilla

Pastry Cream
- ½ cup milk
- ½ tsp vanilla
- Pinch of cornstarch
- 1 tbsp + 1 tsp sugar
- 1 egg yolk
- Optional: powdered sugar, chocolate ganache

Just for Fun Treats

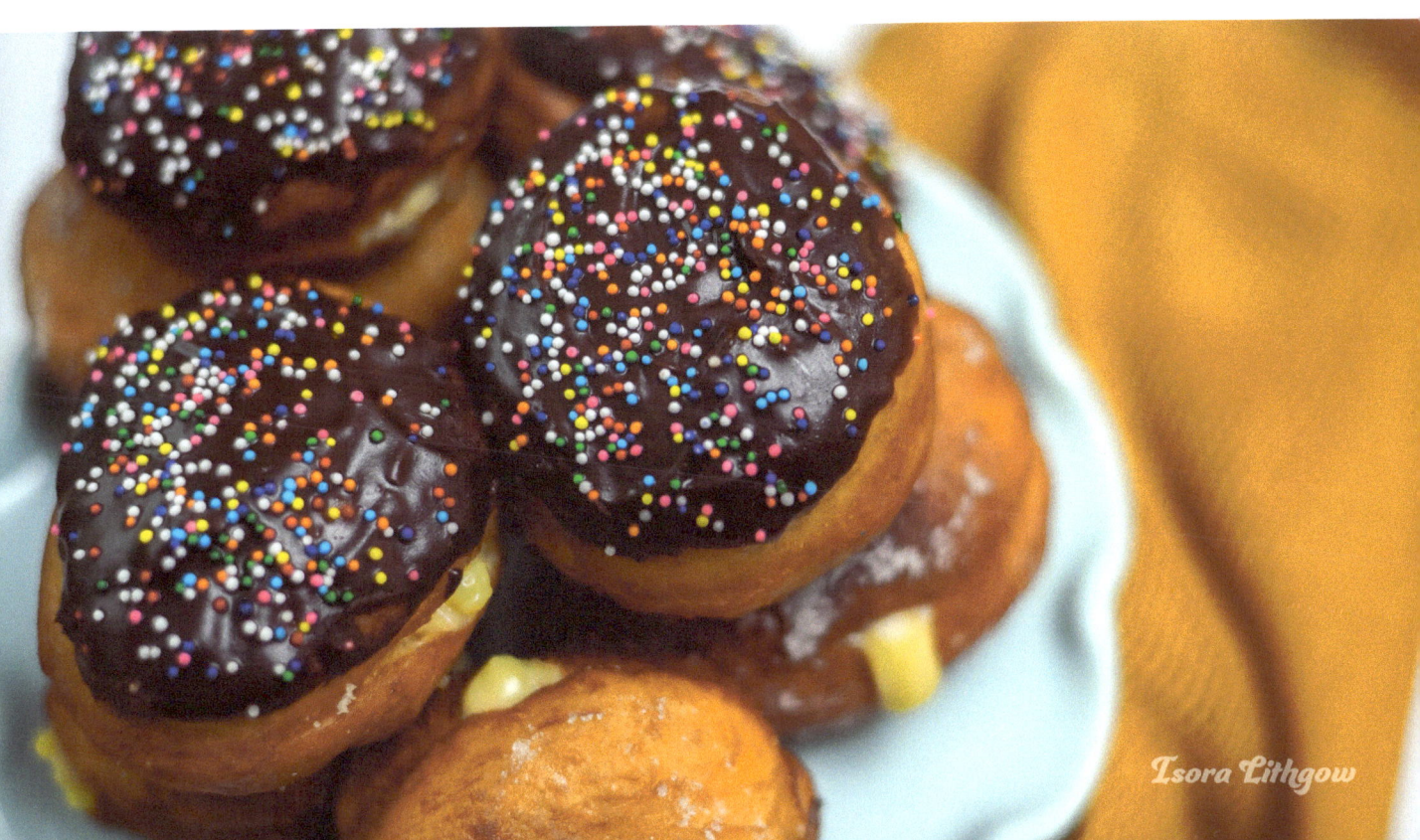

Isora Lithgow

Homemade Peanut Butter Twix Bars

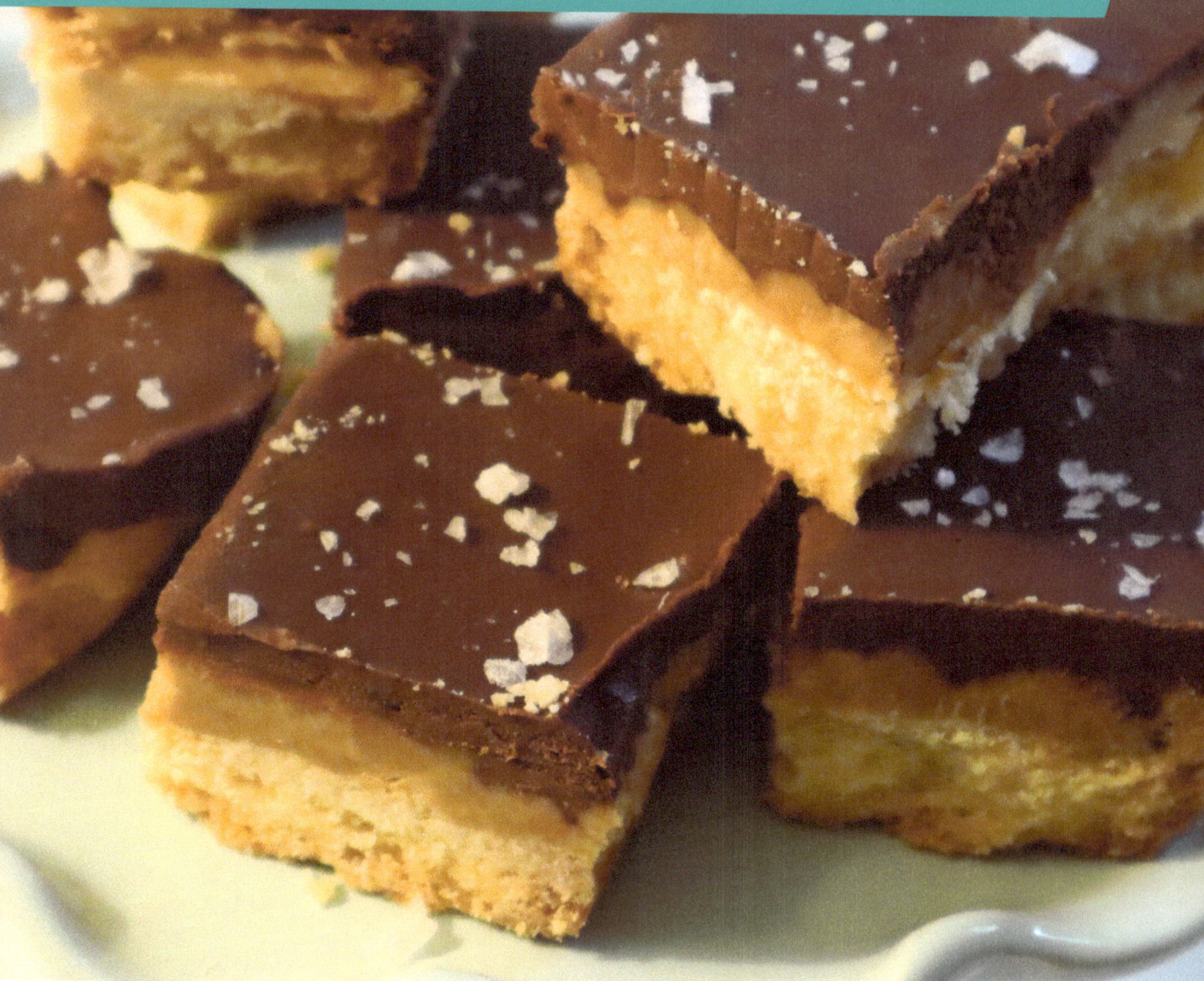

My favorite candy bar is the Peanut Butter Twix—I was so sad when they stopped making them for a few years and thrilled when they reappeared! I prefer the original bar with the shortbread cookie (the reintroduced version has chocolate cookie base) and while these bars aren't quite as neat and pretty looking as the store bought candy bar—they are just as tasty! My philosophy is that how food looks is nice, but taste is everything! The taste here is definitely everything.

Serving:
12 bars

Prep Time:
20 minutes

Bake Time:
35 minutes

Just for Fun Treats

Ingredients

Peanut Butter Filling

- 1 cup peanut butter (creamy)
- ¼ cup butter
- 1 tsp vanilla
- 1 ¼ cups powdered sugar

Chocolate Ganache

- 8 oz chocolate chips
- ¾ cup heavy cream
- 1 tbsp butter

Shortbread Cookie Layer

- 1 ½ sticks unsalted butter, softened
- ½ cup sugar
- 1 tsp vanilla
- 1 ¾ cups flour
- Pinch of salt

Directions

Peanut Butter Filling

1. In a medium saucepan, combine peanut butter, butter, vanilla, and 1 cup of powdered sugar over medium heat.
2. Heat until completely melted and just beginning to bubble, stirring constantly.
3. Remove from heat and slowly stir in remaining powdered sugar until completely combined.
4. Place in fridge to cool while making cookie layer.

Shortbread Cookie Layer

5. Cream butter and sugar, then add vanilla.
6. Mix flour and salt, add to butter mixture and mix on low until loose dough forms.
7. Press dough into a greased square baking pan.
8. Chill in the fridge for about 30 minutes, preheating the oven to 350F.
9. Bake for about 25 minutes, reduce the oven to 325°F and bake for another 10 minutes or until lightly golden.
10. Remove from the oven and cool to room temperature.
11. Spread peanut butter mixture evenly over the shortbread layer and set in the freezer for 15-20 minutes.

Chocolate Ganache

12. Heat heavy cream until about to boil. Pour over chocolate chips and butter and stir until completely melted and shiny.
13. Either cut into squares and carefully dip each cookie piece in the chocolate and coat in a thin layer of chocolate, then place on a wire drying rack to harden.

    OR pour chocolate ganache over top and place in the freezer to set. Once set, cut into squares.

Homemade Peanut Butter Twix Bars

continued

Variations

- Swap peanut butter mixture for caramel for more traditional Twix bars.
- Add sea salt flakes to top before chocolate coating hardens.

Note:
Best stored in the fridge or freezer if not eaten immediately to prevent chocolate and peanut butter from getting too soft and melty.

Double Recipe (24 bars)

Peanut Butter Filling

- 2 cups peanut butter (creamy)
- ½ cup butter
- 2 tsp vanilla
- 2 ½ cups powdered sugar

Chocolate Ganache

- 16 oz chocolate chips
- 1 ½ cups heavy cream
- 2 tbsp butter

Shortbread Cookie Layer

- 3 sticks unsalted butter, softened
- 1 cup sugar
- 2 tsp vanilla
- 3 ½ cups flour
- ¼ tsp of salt

Single Serve (6 bars)

Peanut Butter Filling

- ½ cup peanut butter (creamy)
- 2 tbsp butter
- ½ tsp vanilla
- ½ cup and 2 tbsp powdered sugar

Chocolate Ganache

- 4 oz chocolate chips
- ¼ cup + 2 tbsp heavy cream
- ½ tbsp butter

Shortbread Cookie Layer

- ¾ stick unsalted butter, softened
- ¼ cup sugar
- ½ tsp vanilla
- ¾ cup + 2 tbsp flour
- Pinch of salt

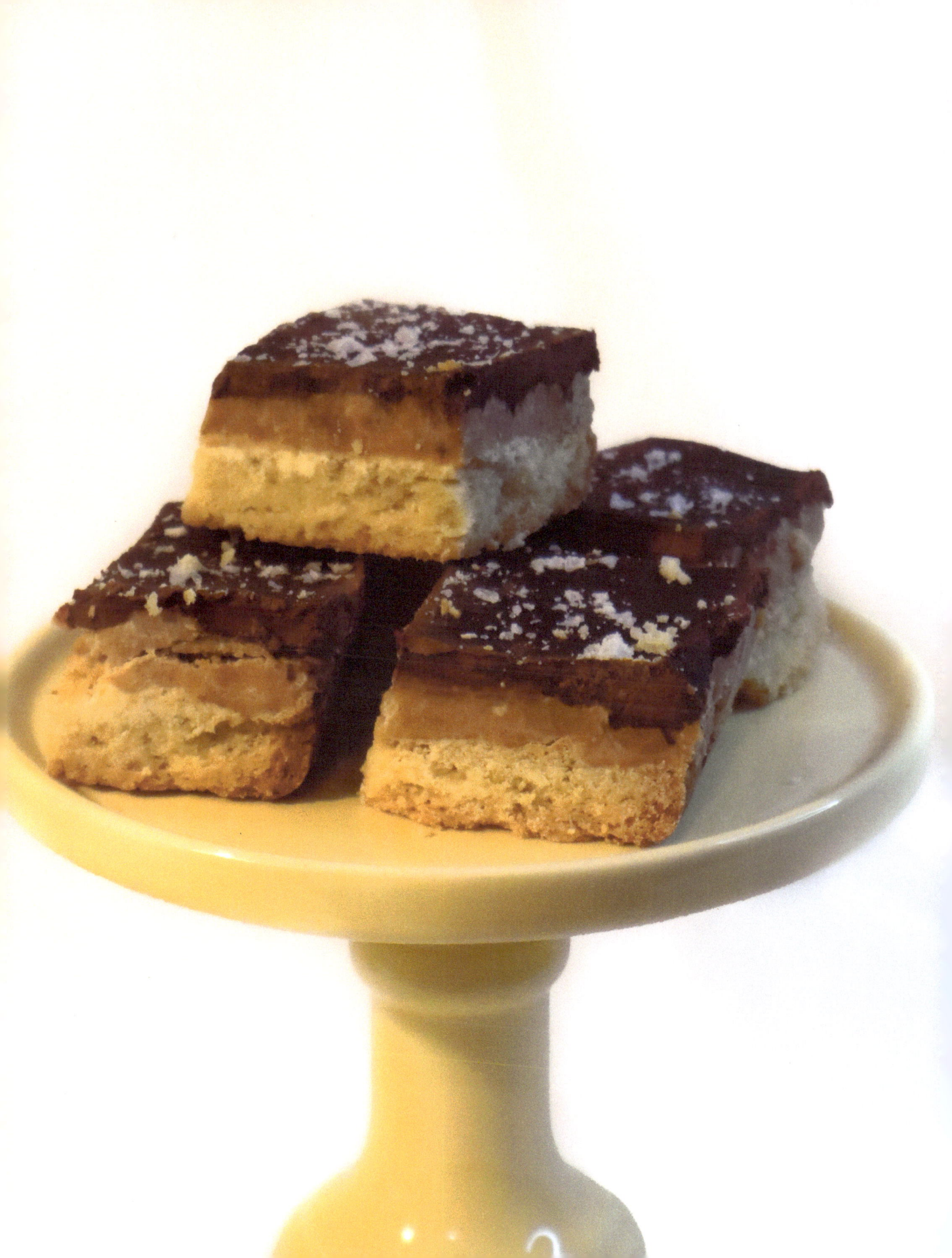

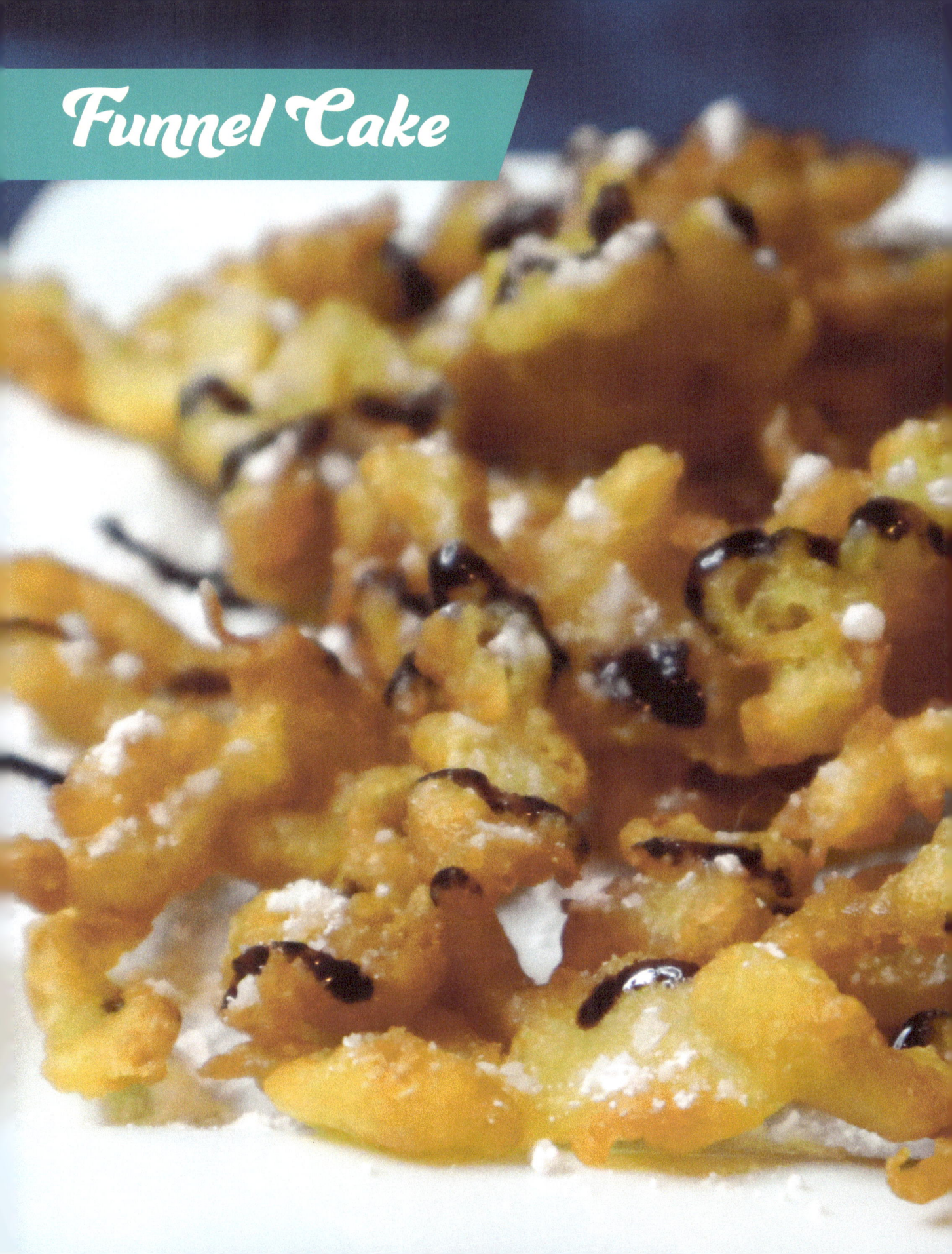

It's funnel cake just like from the fair. It's memories of hot summer days, fair rides until you felt ill, music, playing games for cheap toys, laughing with friends, and filling your belly with deliciously fried fair foods.

Serving:
2 large funnel cakes

Prep Time:
10 minutes

Bake Time:
5 minutes

Ingredients

- ½ cup of milk
- ¼ egg
- ½ tsp of vanilla
- ½ cup of flour
- Pinch of salt
- ¼ tsp baking soda
- ½ tbsp sugar
- 1 ½ tbsp melted butter

Directions

1. In a medium bowl, mix milk, egg, vanilla and butter.
2. Add salt, baking soda and sugar.
3. Slowly fold in flour until batter becomes smooth.
4. Pour batter into a pastry bag and set aside.
5. Heat oil (about an inch deep) in a heavy pan or Dutch oven until it sizzles when you add a drop of water or begins to simmer.
6. Slowly drizzle batter in circles and cook until golden brown on bottom.
7. Gently flip over and cook again until bottom is golden brown.
8. Place on paper towels to drain.
9. Serve with powdered sugar, chocolate, whip cream, etc.
10. Enjoy while fresh and hot!

Double Recipe (4 funnel cakes)

- 1 cup of milk
- ½ egg
- 1 tsp of vanilla
- 1 cup of flour
- Pinch of salt
- ½ tsp baking soda
- 1 tbsp sugar
- 3 tbsp melted butter

Single Serve (1 funnel cake)

- ¼ cup of milk
- ½ tbsp of beaten egg
- ¼ tsp of vanilla
- ¼ cup of flour
- Pinch of salt
- ⅛ tsp baking soda
- 1 tsp sugar
- 1 tbsp melted butter

Just for Fun Treats

Homemade Tootsie Rolls

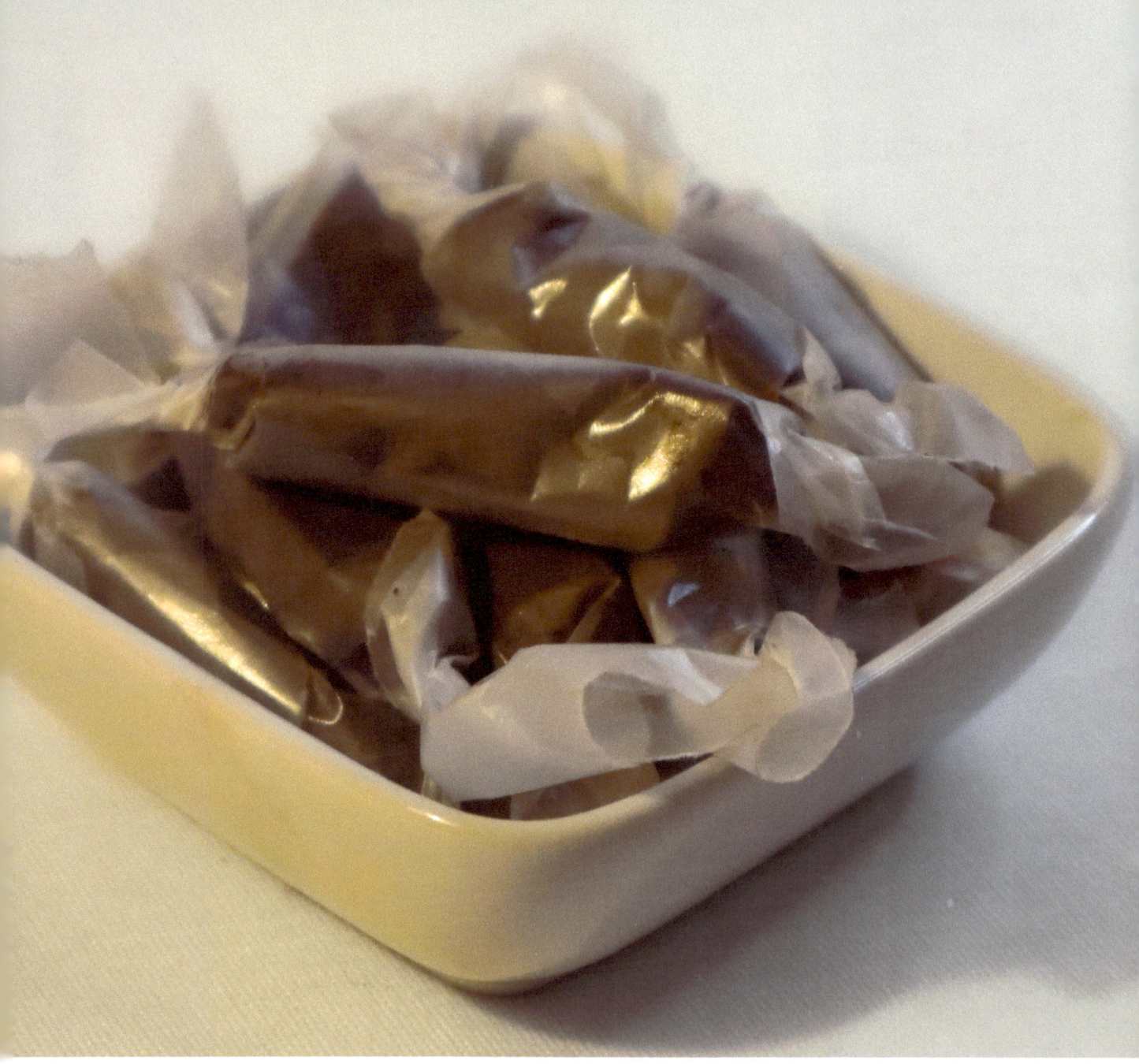

Little bits of chewy chocolate. And shockingly easy to make. Need I say more?

Serving:
24 small rolls

Prep Time:
30 minutes

Bake Time:
none

Just for Fun Treats

Ingredients

- 3 oz chopped milk chocolate (or chocolate chips)
- 3 oz chopped dark chocolate (or chocolate chips)
- ⅔ cup powdered sugar
- ¼ cup light corn syrup
- ⅛ tsp vanilla

Directions

1. Heat milk and dark chocolate on the stove until melted, stirring until smooth.
2. Sift powdered sugar into chocolate and stir until all sugar is dissolved.
3. Continue to stir until slightly cool to touch.
4. Add light corn syrup and vanilla until just combined—do not overmix.
5. Place in a zip top bag and flatten to about ½ inch.
6. Set aside until room temperature, about 1 hour.
7. Remove from the bag and knead until smooth.
8. Break off pieces and roll into ¼ inch ropes.
9. Cut into 3-inch pieces (or 1-inch mini pieces).
10. Wrap in wax paper if desired or store in an airtight container.

Variations

- Can make all milk or dark chocolate if desired.
- Could make peanut butter by replacing chocolate with peanut butter chips.

Note:
Letting chocolate cool slightly before adding corn syrup prevents the final product from becoming greasy.

Double Recipe (48 rolls)

- 6 oz chopped milk chocolate (or chocolate chips)
- 6 oz chopped dark chocolate (or chocolate chips)
- 1⅓ cups powdered sugar
- ½ cup light corn syrup
- ¼ tsp vanilla

Single Serve (12 rolls)

- 1½ oz chopped milk chocolate (or chocolate chips)
- 1½ oz chopped dark chocolate (or chocolate chips)
- ⅓ cup powdered sugar
- 2 tbsp light corn syrup
- ⅛ tsp vanilla

Apple Fritters

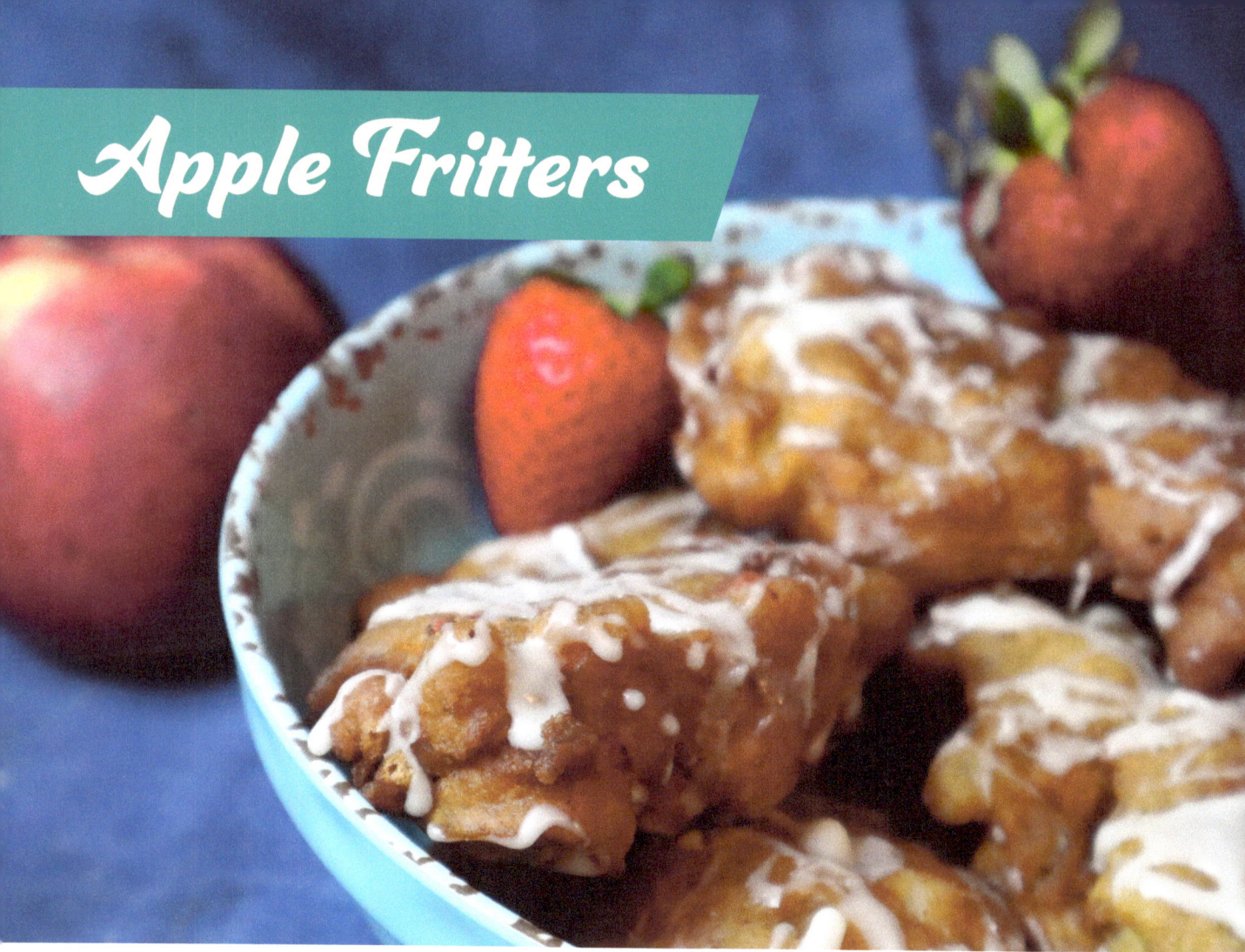

Confession time? I'd never actually eaten an apple fritter before I decided to see if I could make them. But these are my mom's favorite so I decided to give them a try. I have to admit, Mom's got excellent taste! These might be a new favorite for me too.

Serving:
5-6 fritters

Prep Time:
10 minutes

Bake Time:
10 minutes

Ingredients

- ¾ cup flour
- 2 tbsp sugar
- 1 tsp baking powder
- ¼ tsp salt
- ¾ tsp cinnamon
- 3 tbsp + 1 tsp milk
- 1 egg
- 1 ½ tbsp applesauce
- 1 large apple, diced
- Oil for frying

Icing
- 1 cup powdered sugar
- ½ tsp vanilla
- 2 tbsp milk

Directions

1. Whisk together flour, sugar, baking powder, salt and cinnamon.
2. Make a well in center and add milk, egg, and applesauce. Stir to just combine.
3. Fold in diced apples.
4. Heat 1 ½ inch of oil in heavy skillet or Dutch oven (or deep fryer) to 375°F.
5. Drop roughly a ¼ cup of batter at a time into the hot oil, spreading it out as you drop. Fry each side until golden brown.
6. Remove and drain on paper towels.

Icing

7. Whisk together powdered sugar, vanilla, and milk until smooth.
8. Dunk each fritter in icing to coat completely (or drizzle icing on both sides if you prefer less icing). Rest on cooking racks to drip and dry.

Variations

- Strawberries and chocolate chips are a fun substitute for apples.
- Drizzle with chocolate or peanut butter instead of icing.

> **Note:**
> Don't overmix batter or they may become tough.
>
> Best eaten same day but will store wrapped loosely in paper towels in container for a few days.

Double Recipe (10-12 fritters)

- 1 ½ cups flour
- ¼ cup sugar
- 2 tsp baking powder
- ½ tsp salt
- 1 ½ tsp cinnamon
- ⅓ cup milk
- 2 eggs
- 3 tbsp applesauce
- 1-2 large apples, diced
- Oil for frying

Icing

- 2 cups powdered sugar
- 1 tsp vanilla
- ¼ cup milk

Single Serve (2-3 fritters)

- ¼ cup + 2 tbsp flour
- 1 tbsp sugar
- ½ tsp baking powder
- ¼ tsp salt
- ½ tsp cinnamon
- 1 ½ tbsp + ½ tsp milk
- ½ egg
- ¾ tbsp applesauce
- ½ large apple, diced
- Oil for frying

Icing

- ½ cup powdered sugar
- ½ tsp vanilla
- 1 tbsp milk

Fried Pickles

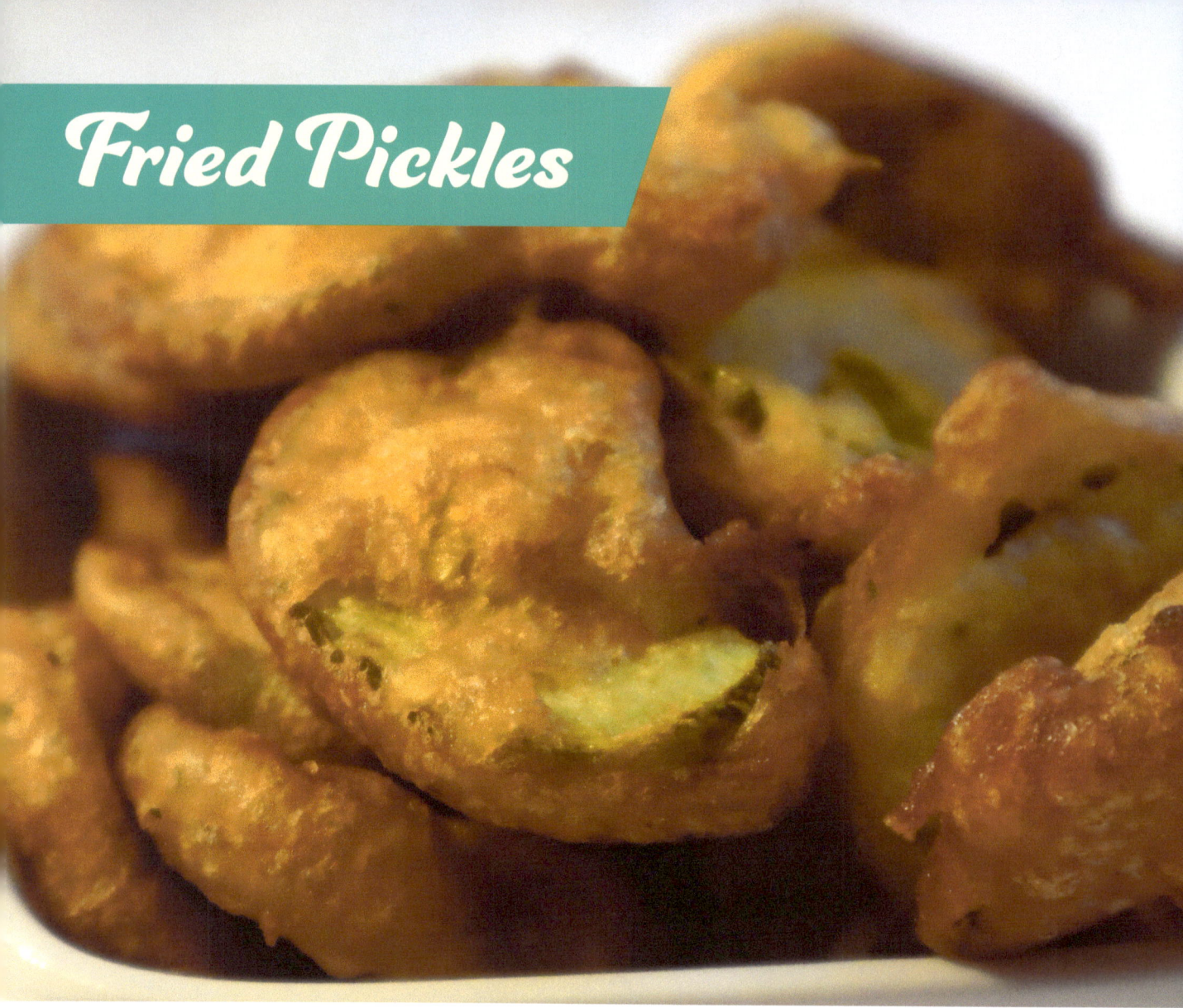

Clearly this pandemic has made me miss my annual excursion for fried fair food! Honestly, the crowds and chaos of fairs have lost their appeal in my adult years, but I have always made it a tradition to go for an hour or two one night, eat all the fair food I could stomach and immediately head home. Absolutely worth the price of admission. Fried pickles are a definite favorite and never missed on my annual excursion! Now I can enjoy them whenever I want in the comfort (and quiet and air conditioning) of my own home. Win-win.

Serving:
4 people

Prep Time:
5 minutes

Bake Time:
15-20 minutes

Ingredients

- 1 cup buttermilk
- ¼ cup milk
- ¾ cup flour
- ½ tsp baking soda
- 1 tsp garlic salt
- 1 tsp parsley
- 1 egg
- 1 jar dill pickle chips/slices
- Canola or vegetable oil for frying

Directions

1. Add all ingredients to a bowl and mix well.
2. Drain pickles and lay out in one layer on a paper towel. Lay another paper towel over top and press to soak up excess pickle juice.
3. Heat oil in a deep fryer and/or in a skillet on the stove until hot. Should sizzle and spit if you drop a water drop into it.
4. Dredge pickle chip through batter to coat with a thin layer and immediately place in oil. Repeat for as many as will fit in the skillet in one layer.
5. Fry until golden brown on bottom (1-3 minutes) and flip to brown on the other side.
6. When fully golden brown, remove and place on a fresh paper towel to drain.
7. When complete, enjoy as is or dip in your favorite dipping sauce!

Just for Fun Treats

Variations

- Can use pickle spears if desired.

Note:

Best to eat fresh!

Any leftover batter can be stored to use later for a few days in the fridge.

Double Recipe (8 people)

- 2 cups buttermilk
- ½ cup milk
- 1 ½ cups flour
- 1 tsp baking soda
- 2 tsp garlic salt
- 2 tsp parsley
- 2 eggs
- 2 jar dill pickle chips/slices
- Canola or vegetable oil for frying

Single Serve (1 person)

- ¼ cup buttermilk
- 1 tbsp milk
- ¼ cup flour
- ⅛ tsp baking soda
- ¼ tsp garlic salt
- ¼ tsp parsley
- ½ egg
- ¼ jar dill pickle chips/slices
- Canola or vegetable oil for frying

Fried Cheese Curds

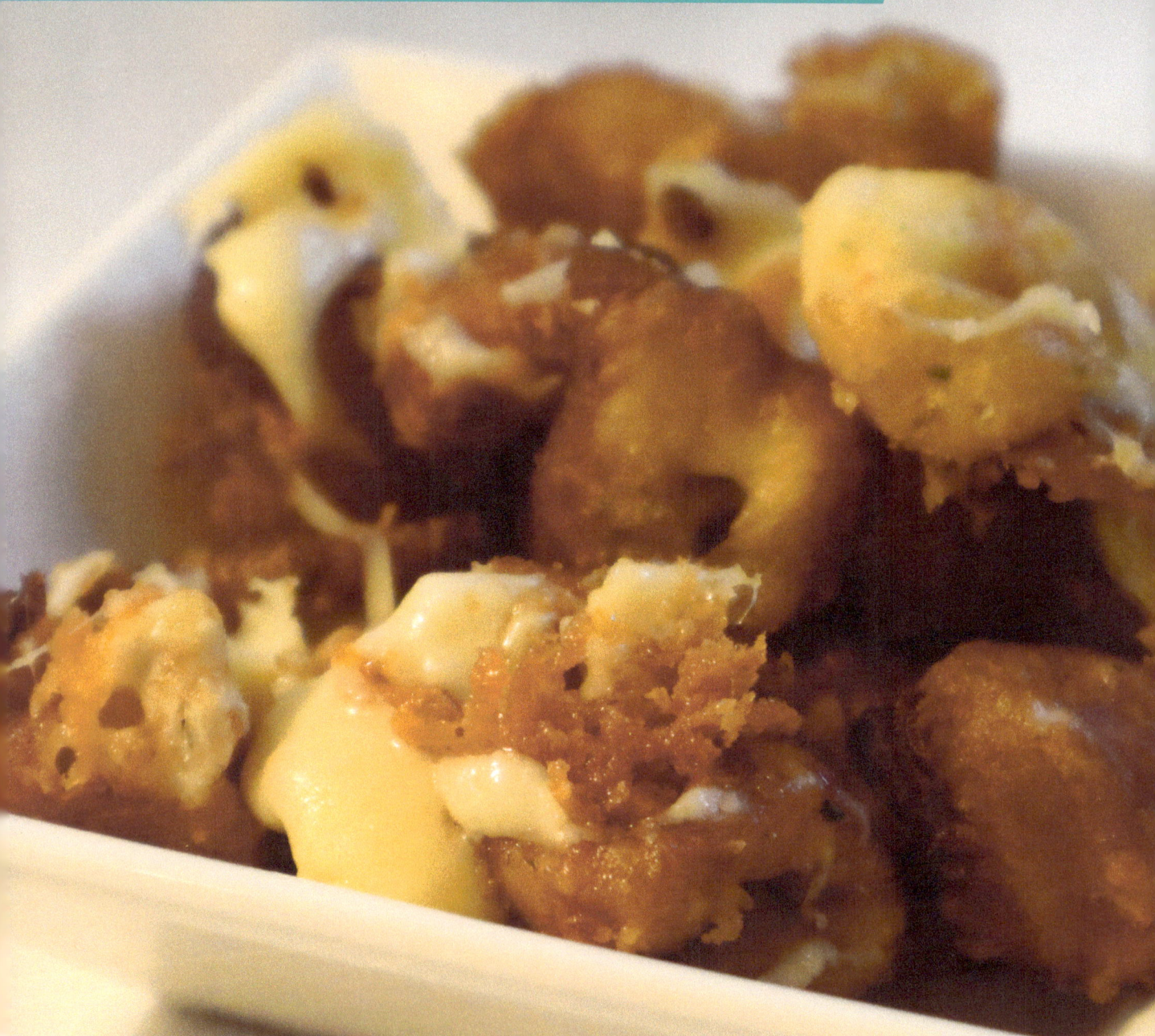

Now these, while also a delicious fair food, are a homage to my roots in Minnesota! Nothing beats genuine cheese curds in Minnesota or Wisconsin—although these are a lovely substitute when one lives across the country. Oozy, gooey cheese encased in batter warms my Midwest farmer daughter's soul.

Serving:
2 people

Prep Time:
5 minutes

Bake Time:
10-15 minutes

Just for Fun Treats

Ingredients

- 1 cup buttermilk
- ¼ cup milk
- ¾ cup flour
- ½ tsp baking soda
- 1 tsp garlic salt
- 1 egg
- 16 oz cheese curds
- Canola or vegetable oil for frying

Directions

1. Add all ingredients to a bowl and mix well.
2. Heat oil in a deep fryer and/or in a skillet on the stove until hot. Should sizzle and spat if you drop a water drop into it.
3. Dredge cheese curd through batter to coat with a thin layer and immediately place in oil. Repeat for as many as will fit in the skillet in one layer.
4. Fry until golden brown on bottom (1-3 minutes) and flip to brown on the other side.
5. When fully golden brown, remove and place on a fresh paper towel to drain.
6. Enjoy the melty, cheesy goodness!

Note:
Best eaten fresh and hot!

Double Recipe (4 people)

- 2 cups buttermilk
- ½ cup milk
- 1 ½ cups flour
- 1 tsp baking soda
- 2 tsp garlic salt
- 2 eggs
- 32 oz cheese curds
- Canola or vegetable oil for frying

Single Serve (1 person)

- ½ cup buttermilk
- 2 tbsp milk
- ¼ cup + 1 tbsp flour
- ¼ tsp baking soda
- ½ tsp garlic salt
- ½ egg
- 8 oz cheese curds
- Canola or vegetable oil for frying

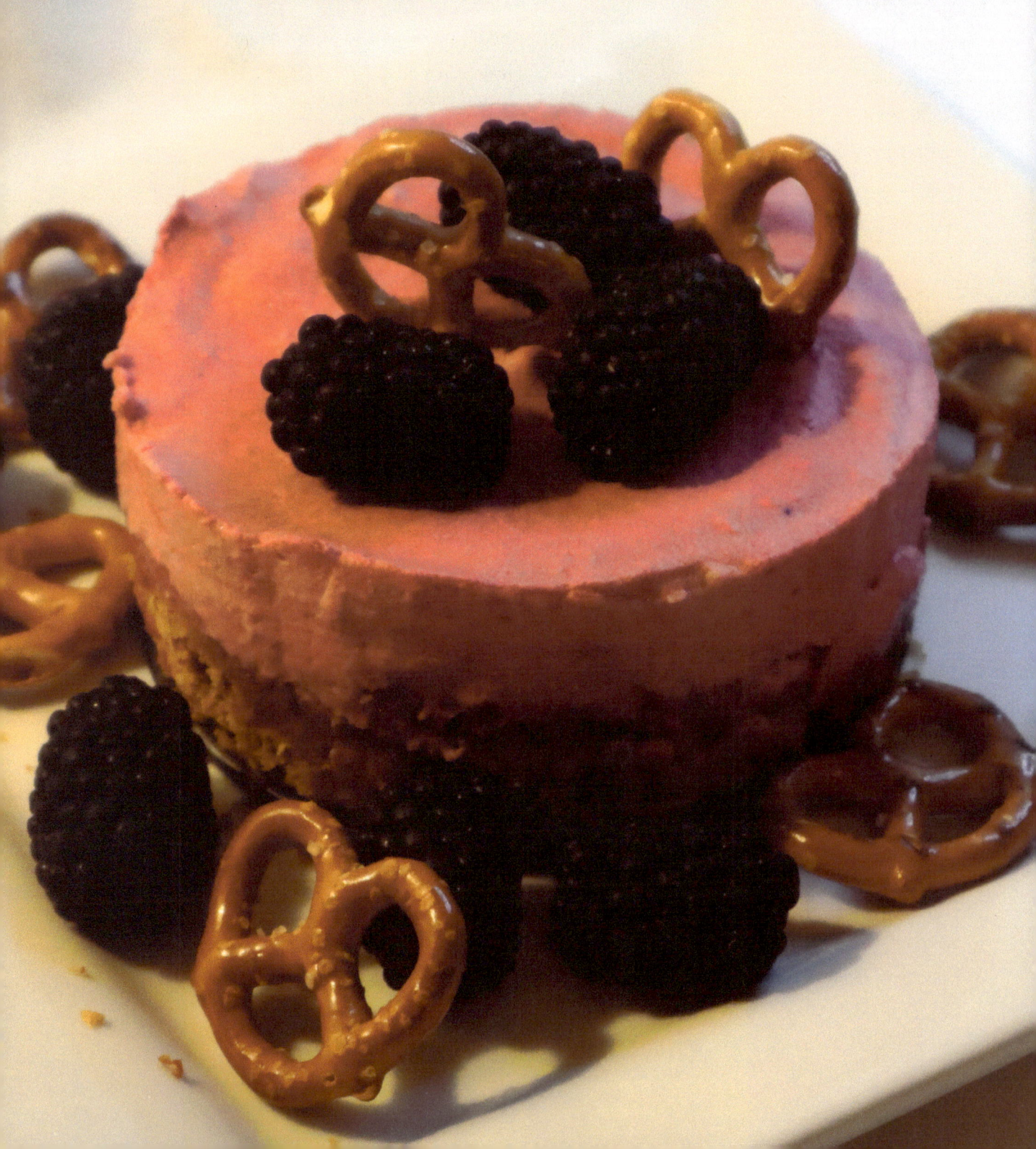

I feel like blackberries are an often forgotten and underrated fruit—juicy and sweet and just a bit tart. Mix that with a salty pretzel crust and it's a delightful combination. The perfect summer dessert.

Serving:
One 10-inch pie

Prep Time:
30 minutes

Bake Time:
10-12 minutes

Ingredients

Crust

- 1 cup crumbled pretzels
- 4 tbsp butter, melted
- 1 tbsp sugar

Mousse

- 1 cup blackberries, fresh or frozen
- ¼ cup sugar
- 1 tbsp powdered sugar
- 1 ½ tbsp milk
- 1 ¼ cups whipping cream
- 1 ½ tsp powdered gelatin
- 1 tbsp water

Directions

Crust

1. Preheat oven to 350°F.
2. Chop pretzels in a food processor until texture of rough sand (10-15 seconds).
3. Add 4 tbsp melted butter and sugar, pulse to combine until it feels like damp sand.
4. Press evenly into the pie pan.
5. Bake for 10-12 minutes. Remove and set aside to cool.

Mousse

6. In small bowl, sprinkle gelatin over water and let sit for 5 minutes.
7. Puree blackberries.
8. Heat blackberry puree with sugar and milk on the stove until just beginning to simmer.
9. Whisk in gelatin until dissolved.
10. Strain through a fine mesh strainer to remove pulp and seeds.
11. Store pulp and seeds for use in other recipes.
12. Whip remaining heavy cream on high until it begins to thicken.
13. Add powdered sugar and whip until stiff peaks form.
14. Fold ⅓ whipped cream into raspberry juice until well combined.
15. Fold in remaining whipped cream.
16. Fill the crust with mousse and place in the fridge to set for at least 2-3 hours.

Blackberry Mousse Pie

continued

Variations

- Can substitute any preferred berries or fruit desired!
- Top with additional whipped cream or pretzel bits.

> **Note:**
> If you don't have a food processor, you can crush pretzels the old fashion way—a rolling pin and zip top bag.

Double Recipe
(two 10-inch pies)

Crust

- 2 cups crumbled pretzels
- 8 tbsp butter, melted
- 2 tbsp sugar

Mousse

- 2 cups blackberries, fresh or frozen
- ½ cup sugar
- 2 tbsp powdered sugar
- 3 tbsp milk
- 2 ½ cups whipping cream
- 3 tsp powdered gelatin
- 2 tbsp water

Single Serve
(one 6-inch pie)

Crust

- ½ cup crumbled pretzels
- 2 tbsp butter, melted
- ½ tbsp sugar

Mousse

- ½ cup blackberries, fresh or frozen
- 2 tbsp sugar
- ½ tbsp powdered sugar
- ¾ tbsp milk
- ½ cup + 2 tbsp whipping cream
- ¾ tsp powdered gelatin
- ½ tbsp water

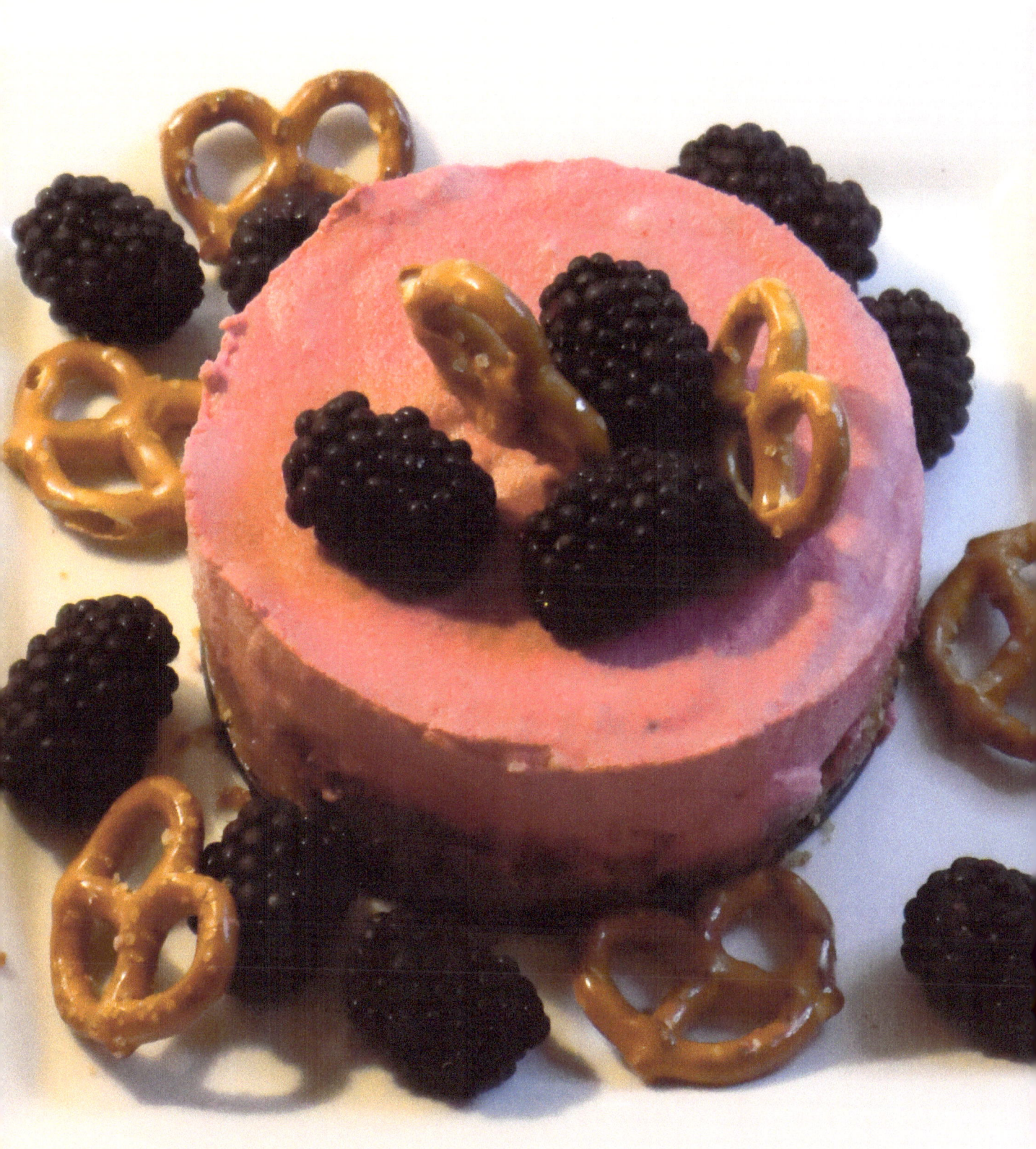

Dark Chocolate Tart

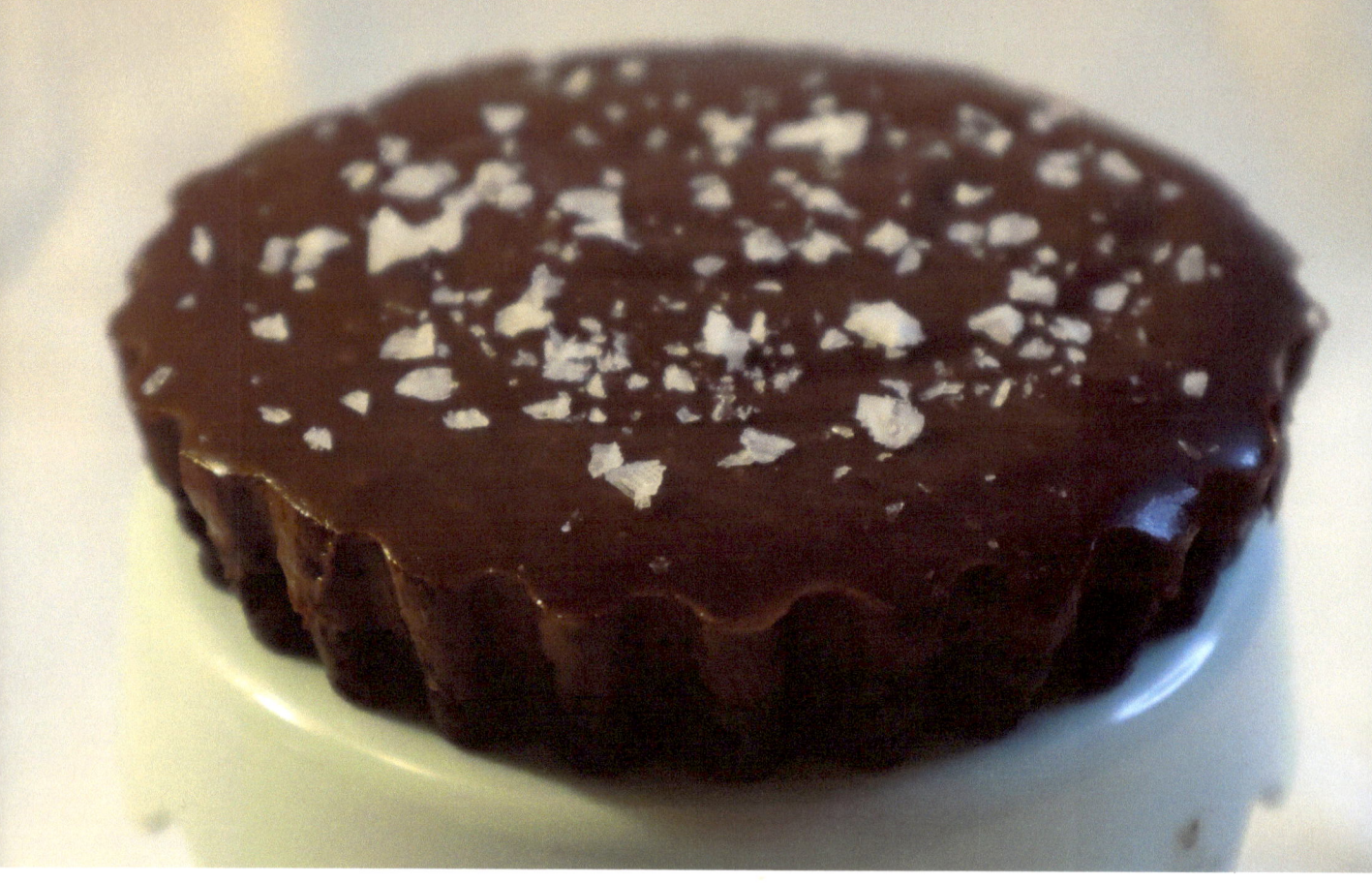

Sheer luscious chocolate bliss. That's all I really have to say about it.

Serving:
12 tarts

Prep Time:
2 hours

Bake Time:
10 minutes

Ingredients

Crust

- 1 ½ cups chocolate wafers (or Oreos), crumbled
- 4 tbsp butter, melted

Ganache

- 1 ½ cups heavy cream
- 12 oz dark chocolate chips
- 4 tbsp butter, room temp
- 1 tbsp flaky sea salt

Whipped Cream

- 1 ½ cups heavy cream
- 1 tsp vanilla
- 1 pinch salt
- ¼ cup powdered sugar

Directions

Crust

1. Preheat oven to 350°F.
2. Grind or crush cookies/wafers and measure out 1 ½ cups.
3. Combine with melted butter until it resembles damp sand.
4. Press crust into a 10-inch tart pan or mini tart pans up the sides, until well packed and even.
5. Bake the crust for 10-12 minutes. Allow to cool.

Ganache

6. Heat heavy cream in a saucepan until just beginning to simmer.
7. Remove from heat and add chocolate chips. Let sit for a few minutes.
8. Whisk cream and chocolate together until smooth and shiny.
9. Add butter, a piece at a time and whisk well.
10. Pour ganache into the prepared tart crust. Place carefully in the refrigerator to set for 2 hours until set. Scatter sea salt across top once set so it doesn't sink into chocolate.

Whipped Cream

11. Whip heavy cream, vanilla, salt, and sugar until medium peaks form.
12. Top tart with whipped cream when ready to serve and enjoy!

Variations

- Can substitute graham cracker or vanilla wafer crumbs for chocolate if desired.

Double Recipe (24 tarts)

Crust

- 3 cups chocolate wafers (or Oreos), crumbled
- 8 tbsp butter, melted

Ganache

- 4 cups heavy cream
- 24 oz dark chocolate chips
- 8 tbsp butter, room temp
- 2 tbsp flaky sea salt

Whipped Cream

- 3 cups heavy cream
- 2 tsp vanilla
- ¼ tsp salt
- ½ cup powdered sugar

Single Serve (6 tarts, mini tart pans or 6-inch crust)

Crust

- ¾ cup chocolate wafers (or Oreos), crumbled
- 2 tbsp butter, melted

Ganache

- ¾ cup heavy cream
- 6 oz dark chocolate chips
- 2 tbsp butter, room temp
- ½ tbsp flaky sea salt

Whipped Cream

- ¾ cup heavy cream
- ½ tsp vanilla
- 1 pinch salt
- 2 tbsp powdered sugar

Blueberry Hand Pies

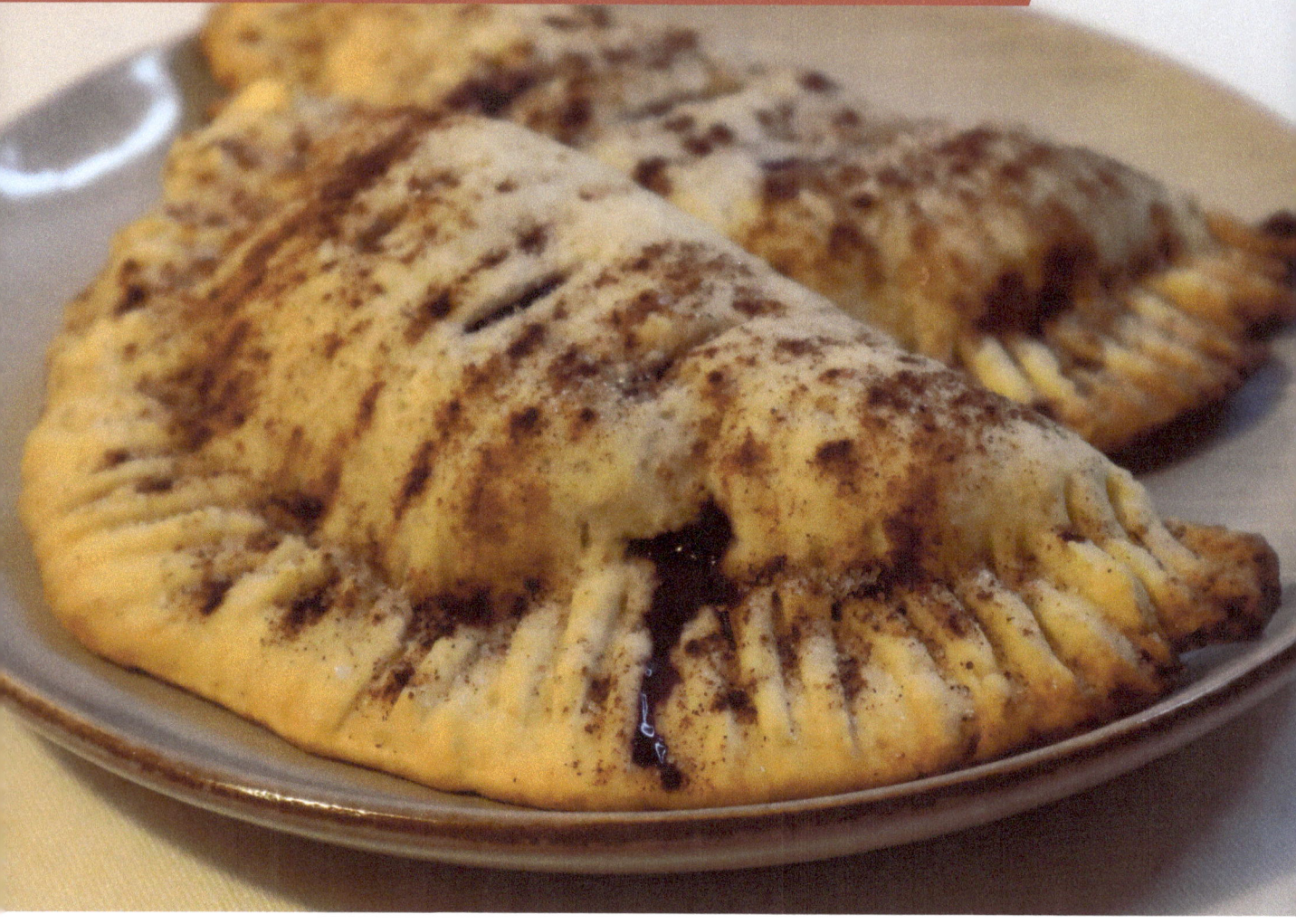

This is one recipe in which I pull from my Midwestern church cookbook roots and tell you to get a store bought pie crust—convenience is highly valued in practical Midwestern church ladies who rely heavily on store bought pie crusts and frozen bread dough. One of these days I'll get the hang of homemade pie crusts! Whether homemade or store bought crusts—it's pie, bursting with blueberry goodness, that you can hold in your hand. What could be better? Serve with a scoop of ice cream for maximum enjoyment.

Serving:
4 hand pies

Prep Time:
15 minutes

Bake Time:
10 minutes

Ingredients

- 1 cup blueberries (fresh or frozen)
- 1 tbsp sugar
- 1 tsp cinnamon
- 1 tsp cornstarch
- 1 ½ tsp vanilla
- 1 pie crust (homemade or store bought)

Directions

1. Preheat the oven to 425°F.
2. Mix blueberries, sugar, cinnamon, cornstarch and vanilla in a saucepan on medium heat.
3. Heat until blueberries release their juices.
4. Reduce heat to low and simmer until thickens.
5. Remove from heat.
6. Divide pie crust into 4 equal parts on a baking sheet.
7. Drop approximately 1 to 2 tbsp blueberry mixture into each piece.
8. Fold crust over and press edges together with fingers to seal. If possible, fold edges back on themselves to further seal and prevent leakage.
9. Crimp edges of hand pie with fork and cut 3-4 small slits on top (or use fork to poke 5-6 times).
10. Sprinkle tops with cinnamon sugar.
11. Bake for about 10 minutes or until golden brown on edges.
12. Cool for 5-10 minutes and enjoy!

Variations

- Substitute any preferred fruit for blueberries.

Double Recipe (8 hand pies)

- 2 cups blueberries (fresh or frozen)
- 2 tbsp sugar
- 2 tsp cinnamon
- 2 tsp cornstarch
- 3 tsp vanilla
- 2 pie crusts (homemade or store bought)

Single Serve (2 hand pies)

- ½ cup blueberries (fresh or frozen)
- ½ tbsp sugar
- ½ tsp cinnamon
- ½ tsp cornstarch
- 1 tsp vanilla
- ½ pie crust (homemade or store bought)

Cheesy Pesto & Asparagus Tart

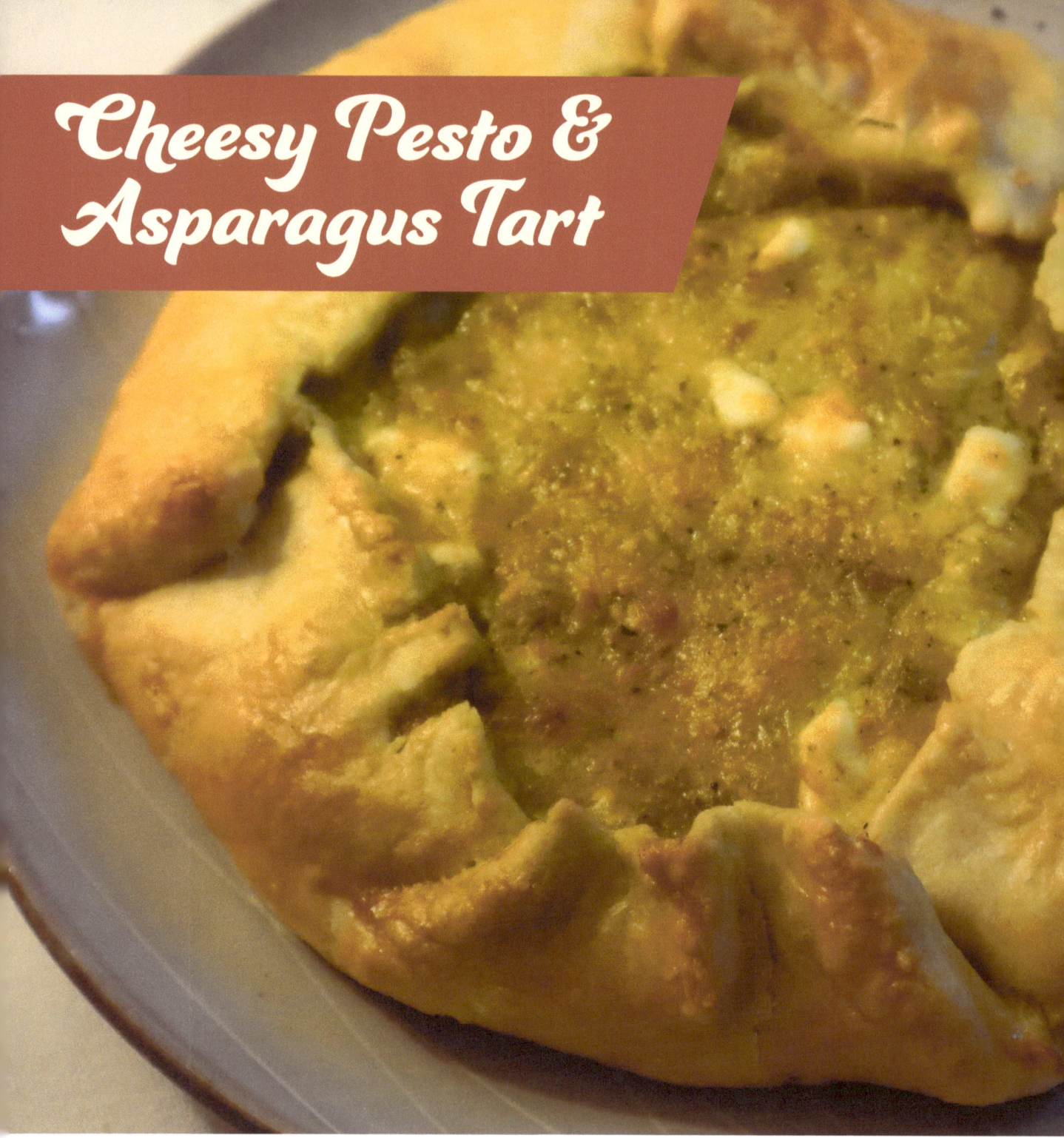

I will never tire of finding different ways to combine eggs, cheese, pesto and various kinds of bread and/or crusts. This savory wonder cradled in flaky crust is a definite must. Topped with asparagus—my favorite veggie of all—tips it into a world class winner category. If I can't eat pizza every day, this is a lovely alternative!

Serving:
2 tarts

Prep Time:
1 hour, 10 minutes

Bake Time:
25 minutes

Ingredients

Crust
- 1 ½ cups flour
- ¾ tsp salt
- ¼ cup shortening
- ¼ cup butter
- ¼ cup + 1 tbsp ice cold water

Filling
- ¾ cup mozzarella cheese
- ½ cup feta cheese
- 1 egg
- Splash of milk
- ½ tsp salt
- 1 ½ tbsp pesto
- 6-7 asparagus stalks
- 1 beaten egg (for brushing on crust)

Directions

Crust
1. Mix together flour and salt. Cut in shortening and butter with a pastry blender (or use a food processor) until pea-sized crumbs.
2. Sprinkle cold water over mixture, a little at a time, stirring with fork until dough forms a loose ball. Chill dough for about an hour to help with rolling out.
3. Preheat the oven to 400°F.

Filling
4. Combine cheeses, egg, splash of milk, salt, and pesto together.
5. Divide dough into 2 equal pieces. Roll each out into a roughly 8-inch round.
6. Spoon filling into the middle of each dough round, leaving about 2 inches of crust around the edge.
7. Top with 3-4 two inches of asparagus.
8. Gently fold the edge of the crust over filling, pleating as you go. Brush the crust with beaten egg. Bake for 25-30 minutes or until the crust is golden brown and cheesy egg mixture is baked through.
9. Enjoy warm!

Variations
- Can substitute for preferred cheeses or veggies.
- Melty brie cheese would be a decadent substitution.
- Substitute tomato sauce for pesto.
- Add herbs to taste.

Note:
Dough can be made in a food processor for ease.

Pies & Tarts

Cheesy Pesto & Asparagus Tart

continued

Double Recipe (4 tarts)

Crust
- 3 cups flour
- 1 ½ tsp salt
- ½ cup shortening
- ½ cup butter
- ½ cup + 1 tbsp ice cold water

Filling
- 1 ½ cups mozzarella cheese
- 1 cup feta cheese
- 2 eggs
- Splash of milk
- 1 tsp salt
- 3 tbsp pesto
- 12-14 asparagus stalks
- 1 beaten egg (for brushing on crust)

Single Serve (1 tart)

Crust
- ¾ cup flour
- ¼ tsp salt
- 2 tbsp shortening
- 2 tbsp butter
- 2 tbsp + 1 tsp ice cold water

Filling
- ½ cup mozzarella cheese
- ¼ cup feta cheese
- 1 egg
- Splash of milk
- ¼ tsp salt
- 1 tbsp pesto
- 3-4 asparagus stalks
- 1 beaten egg (for brushing on crust)

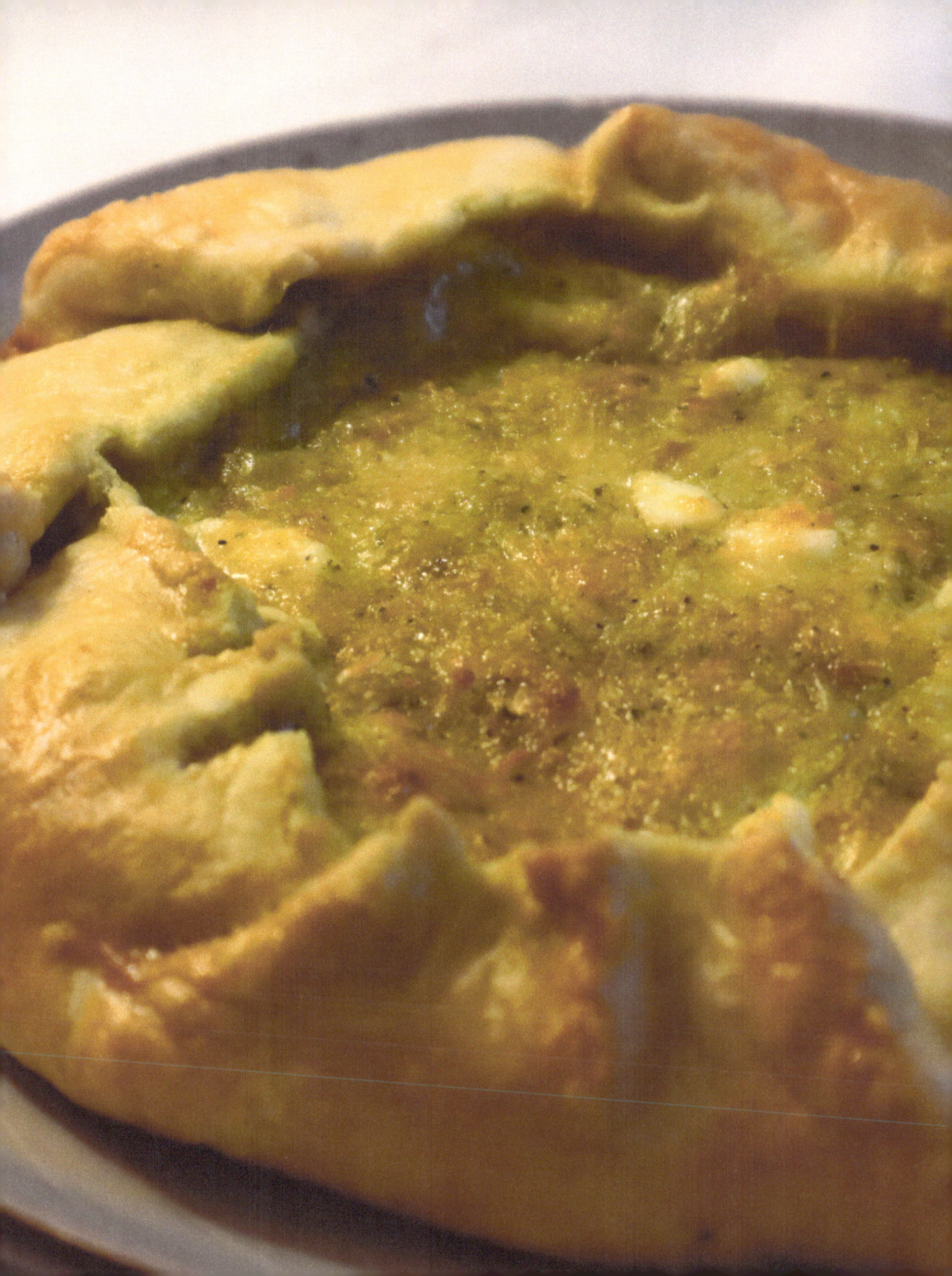

Chocolate Cream Pie with Sugar Cookie Crust

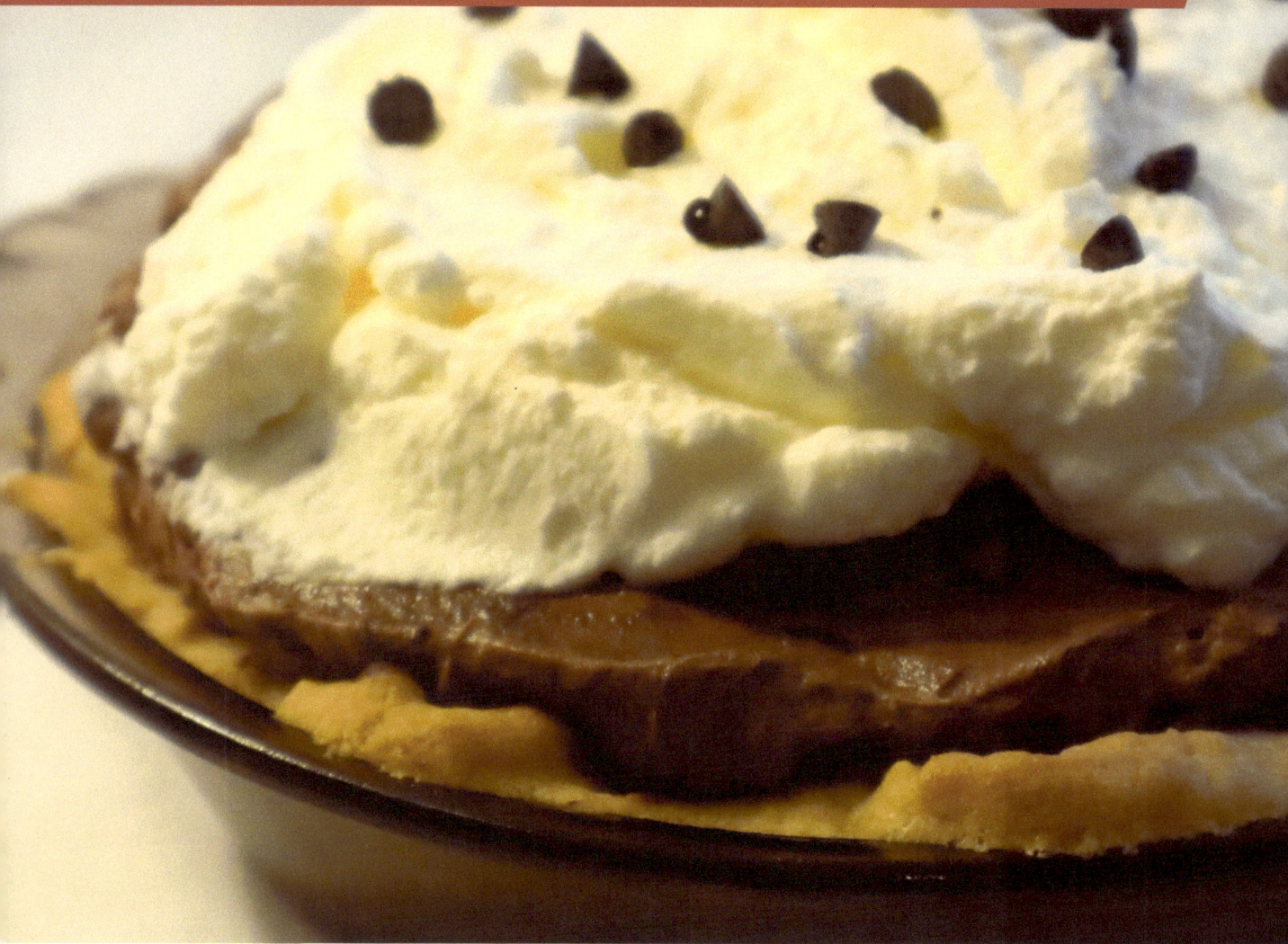

Chocolate Cream filling in a **sugar cookie** crust. The ultimate dessert for those with a sweet tooth. Enjoy the sugar rush!

Serving:
6-inch pie pan

Prep Time:
4 hours, 15 minutes

Bake Time:
20-25 minutes

Ingredients

Crust
- 6 tbsp butter, room temp
- ¼ cup + 2 tbsp packed brown sugar
- 1 tsp vanilla
- ½ egg, room temp
- 1 cup flour
- ¼ tsp baking soda
- ¼ tsp salt
- 2 oz chocolate chips
- 1 tsp coconut oil

Whipped Cream
- 2 cups whipping cream
- ⅓ cup powdered sugar

Chocolate Cream Filling
- 2 tbsp butter
- 3 oz semisweet chocolate chips
- ¾ cup powdered sugar
- ¼ cup cocoa powder
- 4 oz softened cream cheese
- 1 ½ cups prepared whipped cream (remainder on top)

Directions

1. Preheat the oven to 350°F.

Crust

2. Cream together the butter and brown sugar until light and fluffy.
3. Add vanilla and egg, mix until combined.
4. Add flour, baking soda, and salt, beat until combined and starts to form a rough ball.
5. Roll out the dough on a floured surface to about ¼ in thickness and 1 inch wider around than the pie pan.
6. Transfer carefully to the greased pie pan and press until it lays flat and even. Poke bottom with fork 10-12 times.
7. In the meantime, place the crust in the freezer for 10-20 minutes. (This will help it hold its shape.)
8. Bake for 10-13 minutes or until just browned. Bottom may look slightly puffy and not quite done.
9. Melt chocolate chips and coconut oil and stir until smooth. Brush over the crust to coat and set in the fridge to cool and harden. (This helps keep cookie crust from getting soggy.)

Whipped Cream

10. While crust bakes, whip whipping cream and powdered sugar on high for about 5-7 minutes until stiff peaks form.
11. Move to the fridge to chill until needed.

Chocolate Cream Filling

12. Cream together cream cheese, powdered sugar, and cocoa powder until smooth.
13. Melt chocolate chips and butter in a small dish in 30 second intervals in the microwave (or on the stove) and stir until smooth.
14. Add melted chocolate and whipped cream to the creamed mix and blend until smooth.
15. Once the crust is cool, fill with chocolate cream filling and top with remaining whipped cream. Add chocolate shavings if desired. Chill in the fridge for 4+ hours before serving.

Note:
Make sure butter and cream cheese are softened before mixing so that it mixes smooth.

Chocolate Cream Pie with Sugar Cookie Crust

continued

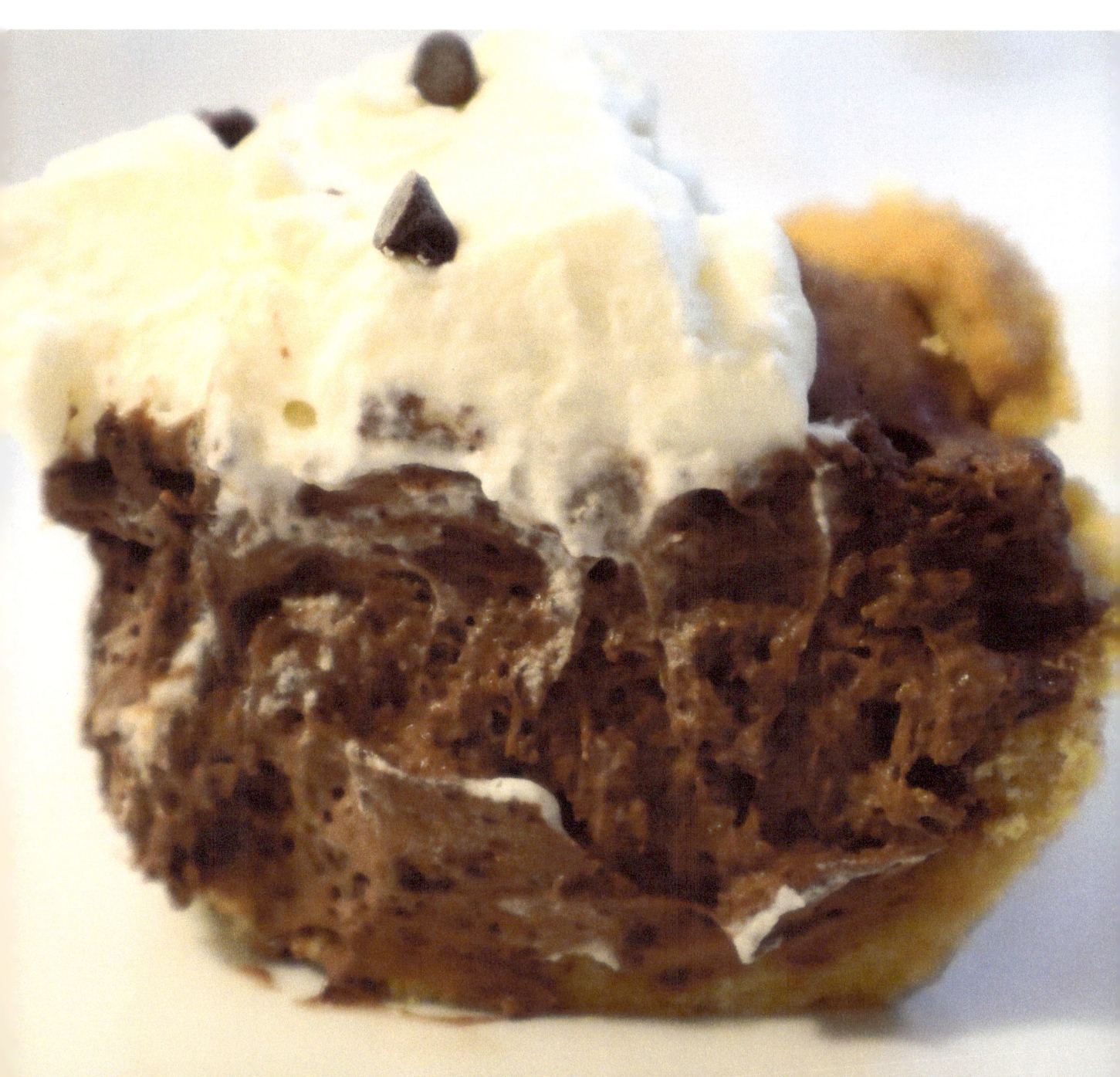

Variations

- Swap chocolate chips for 5 oz peanut butter chocolate chips or creamy PB (and leave out cocoa powder) for peanut butter pie.
- Add a ¼ cup cocoa powder to make chocolate whipped cream (mix with powdered sugar) for double chocolate cream pie.

Double Recipe
(9-10-inch pie)

Crust
- 1 ½ sticks (¾ cup) butter, room temp
- ¾ cup packed brown sugar
- 2 tsp vanilla
- 1 egg, room temp
- 2 cups flour
- ½ tsp baking soda
- ½ tsp salt

Whipped Cream
- 3 cups whipping cream
- ⅓ rounded cup powdered sugar

Chocolate Cream Filling
- 4 tbsp butter
- 6 oz semisweet chocolate chips
- 1 ½ cups powdered sugar
- ½ cup cocoa powder
- 8 oz softened cream cheese
- 3 cups prepared whipped cream (remainder on top)

Single Serve
(4-inch mini pie)

Crust
- 3 tbsp butter, room temp
- 3 tbsp packed brown sugar
- ½ tsp vanilla
- ⅓ egg, room temp
- ½ cup flour
- ⅛ tsp baking soda
- ⅛ tsp salt

Whipped Cream
- 1 cup whipping cream
- ¼ cup powdered sugar

Chocolate Cream Filling
- 1 tbsp butter
- 1 ½ oz semisweet chocolate chips
- ½ cup and 2 tbsp powdered sugar
- 2 tbsp cocoa powder
- 2 oz softened cream cheese
- ¾ cup prepared whipped cream (remainder on top)

Raspberry & Vanilla Cream Tarts

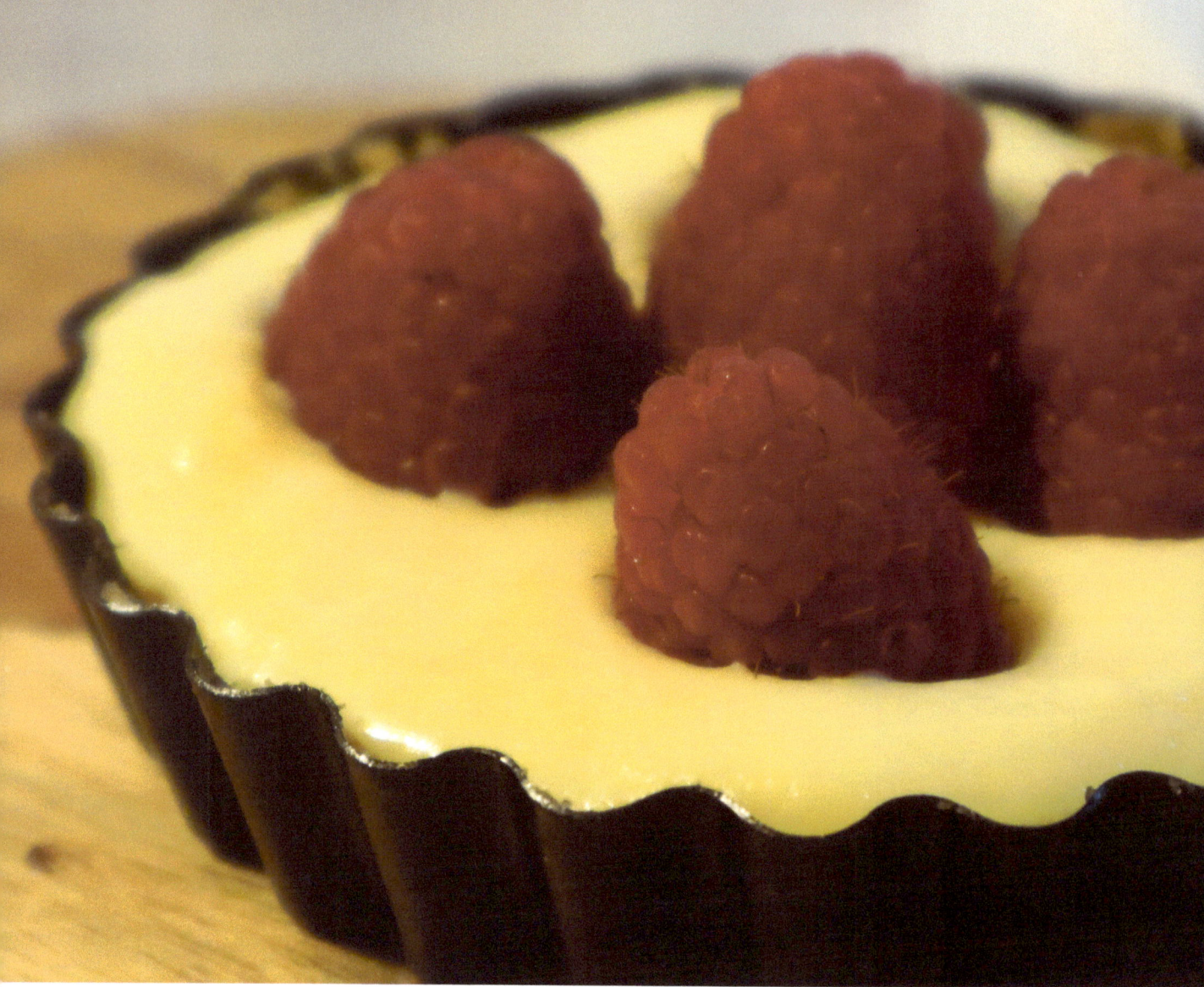

Light and sweet, a perfect summer treat. I am not a summer person—I was built for snow and cold and hot cocoa by the fire. However, summer redeems itself with its abundance of amazing fresh fruits. Raspberries are a particular favorite of mine. These tarts are a lovely reason to eat more of them.

Serving:
5 mini tarts

Prep Time:
30 minutes

Bake Time:
15-20 minutes

Ingredients

Crust
- ¾ cup + 1 tbsp flour
- ¼ cup + 1 tbsp sugar
- Pinch of salt
- ¼ cup butter, cubed
- ½ egg yolk

Vanilla Pastry Cream
- 2 cups milk
- 1 tsp vanilla
- ¼ tsp cornstarch
- ¼ cup + 1 tbsp sugar
- 2 egg yolk

Topping
- Raspberries

Directions

Crust
1. Preheat oven to 400°F.
2. In food processor, blend flour, sugar, and salt for about 10 seconds.
3. Add cubed butter and process until becomes coarse crumbs.
4. Add egg yolk and process again until the egg is thoroughly combined.
5. Press dough into tart molds, making sides slightly higher than the center.
6. Bake for approximately 12-15 minutes, pricking with a fork at intervals to prevent dough from puffing up. Watch carefully as it can become overdone quickly!

Vanilla Cream
7. Combine 1 ½ cups milk and vanilla in a medium saucepan. Cook over high heat until just beginning to simmer, stirring often. Remove from heat.
8. In a medium bowl, whisk remaining milk, egg yolk, sugar, and cornstarch.
9. While whisking vigorously, slowly pour hot milk into the egg mixture.
10. Return mixture to saucepan and cook, continuously whisking until it thickens and begins to boil.
11. Place plastic wrap directly on top of pastry cream to prevent a skin from forming.
12. Cool to room temperature, then place in the fridge for 2-3 hours to set. Whip before use.
13. Put ¼ – ⅓ cup vanilla cream into each cooled crust.
14. Top with raspberries and serve!

Raspberry & Vanilla Cream Tarts

continued

Variations

- Add a drizzle of melted chocolate or chocolate shavings to top.
- Exchange raspberries for your fruit of choice.
- Add a dusting of sparkling sugar or sprinkles for a bit of fun.

Double Recipe
(10 mini tarts)

Crust

- 1 ⅓ cups flour
- ⅓ cup sugar
- Pinch of salt
- ½ cup butter, cubed
- 1 egg yolk

Vanilla Pastry Cream

- 4 cups milk
- 2 tsp vanilla
- ½ tsp cornstarch
- ½ cup + 2 tbsp sugar
- 4 egg yolk

Topping

- Raspberries

Single Serve
(2 mini tarts)

Crust

- ¼ cup + 2 tbsp flour
- 2 ½ tbsp sugar
- Pinch of salt
- 2 tbsp butter, cubed
- ¼ egg yolk

Vanilla Pastry Cream

- 1 cup milk
- ½ tsp vanilla
- ⅛ tsp of cornstarch
- 2 tbsp + 2 tsp sugar
- 1 egg yolk

Topping

- Raspberries

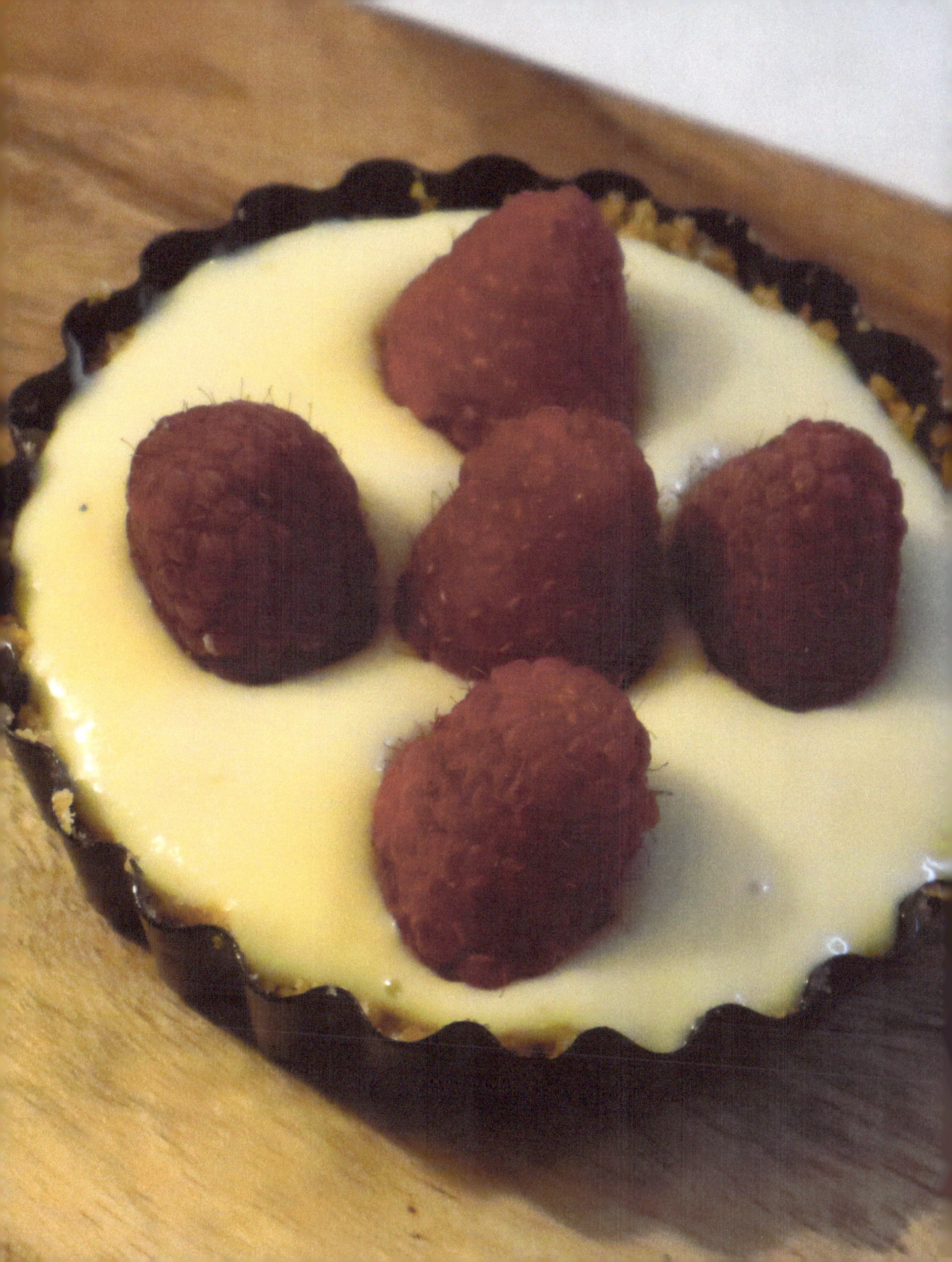

Rustic Peach Tart

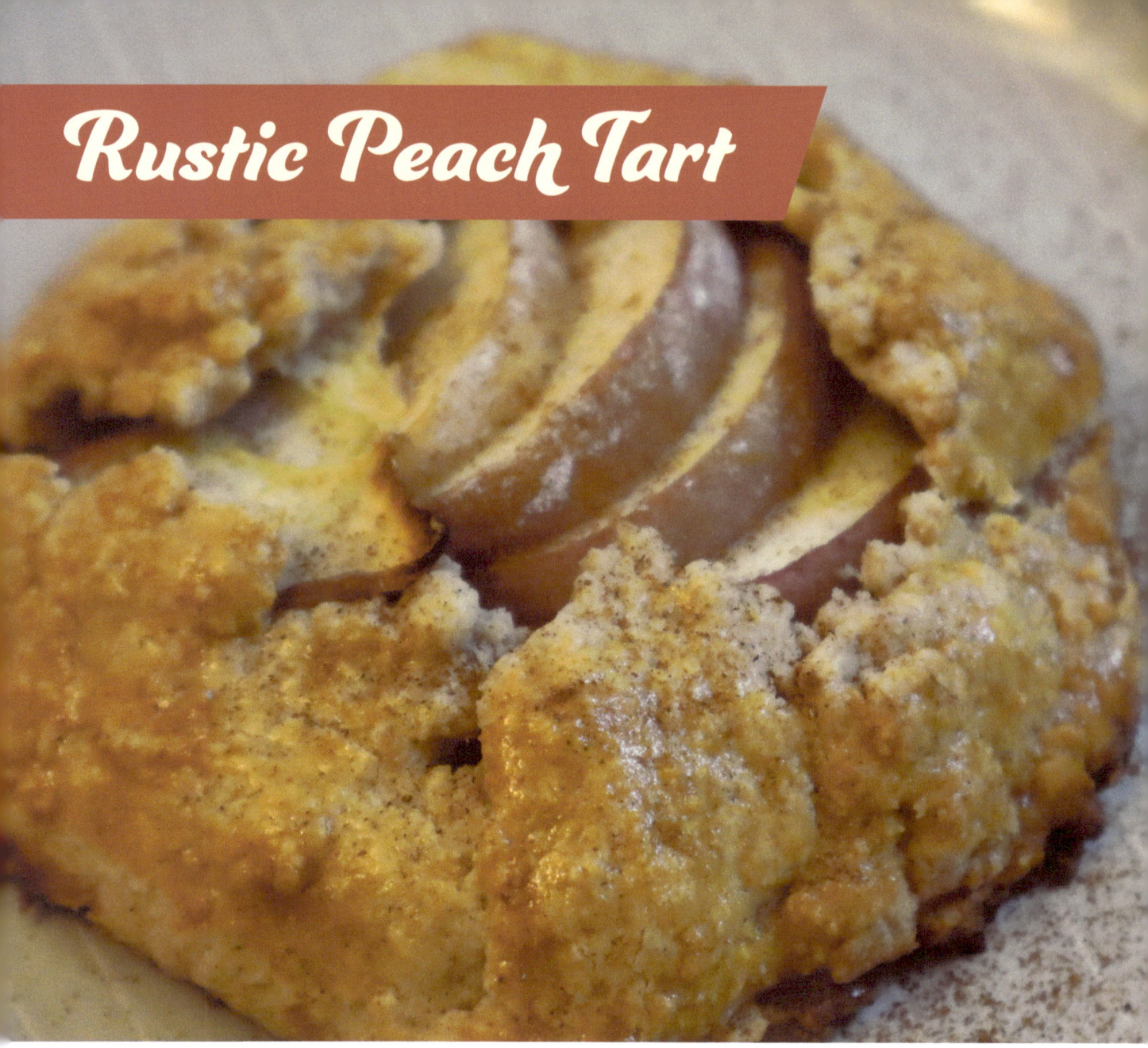

If I'm being honest, I tend to buy fresh peaches in the summer when I see them and then promptly forget about them in the fridge. Oops. These tarts came about as a tasty solution to my peach problem! My fading peaches were saved when baked in a flaky crust and enjoyed for breakfast (and a few snacks). They don't always look pretty when I make them, but they always taste like summer sunshine.

Serving:
2 tarts

Prep Time:
1 hour, 10 minutes

Bake Time:
25 minutes

Ingredients

Crust
- 1 ½ cups flour
- ¾ tsp salt
- 2 tbsp sugar
- 1 tsp cinnamon
- ½ cup shortening
- ¼ cup + 1 tbsp ice cold water

Filling
- 2-3 sliced peaches (fresh or frozen)
- 3 tbsp sugar
- 1 ½ tsp cornstarch
- 1 beaten egg (for brushing the crust)

Variations
- Can substitute mangos, berries, apples, etc. for peaches as desired.

Directions

Crust
1. Mix together flour, salt, and sugar. Cut in shortening with a pastry blender (or by hand) until pea-sized crumbs.
2. Sprinkle cold water over mixture, stirring with fork until dough forms a loose ball. Chill dough for about an hour to help with rolling out.
3. Preheat the oven to 400°F.

Filling
4. Toss peach slices with sugar and cornstarch.
5. Divide dough into 2 equal pieces. Roll each out into a roughly 8-inch round.
6. Layer peach slices in the middle of each dough round, leaving about an inch & a half of crust around the edge.
7. Gently fold the edge of the crust over peaches, pleating as you go. Brush the crust with beaten egg. Bake for 25-30 minutes or until the crust is golden brown and the peaches are tender.

Double Recipe (4 tarts)

Crust
- 3 cups flour
- 1 ½ tsp salt
- 4 tbsp sugar
- 2 tsp cinnamon
- 1 cup shortening
- ½ cup + 2 tbsp ice cold water

Filling
- 3-6 sliced peaches (fresh or frozen)
- 6 tbsp sugar
- 3 tsp cornstarch
- 1 beaten egg (for brushing the crust)

Single Serve (1 tart)

Crust
- ¾ cup flour
- ¼ tsp salt
- 1 tbsp sugar
- ½ tsp cinnamon
- ¼ cup shortening
- 1 tbsp + 1 tsp ice cold water

Filling
- 1-2 sliced peaches (fresh or frozen)
- 1 ½ tbsp sugar
- ¾ tsp cornstarch
- 1 beaten egg (for brushing the crust)

Sonya's Raspberry Lemonade

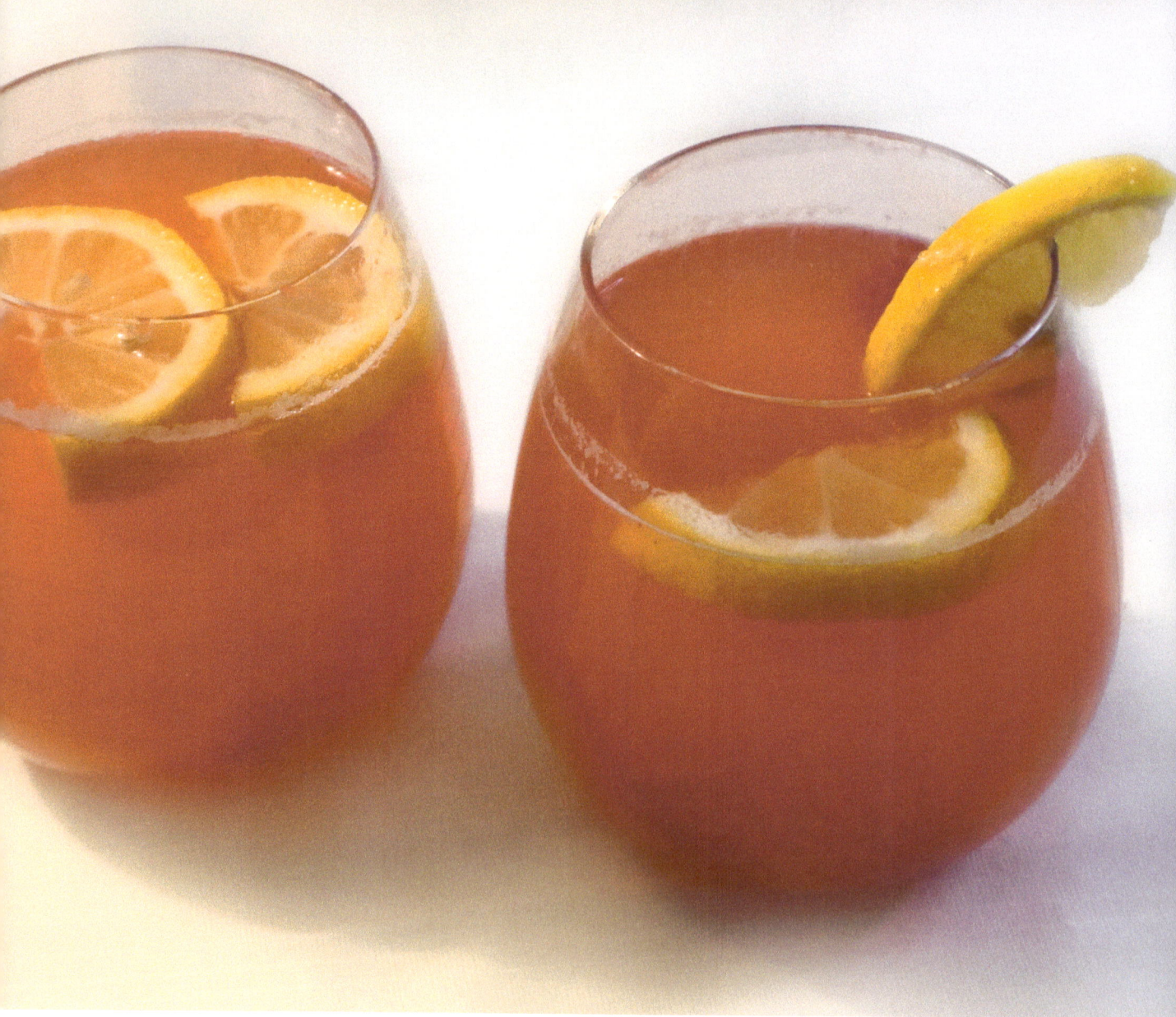

A sweet and tart treat for summer inspired by a young friend named Sonya. Her talk of fruity lemonade wouldn't get out of my head until I decided to try my hand at making my own homemade lemonade—with a fruity twist. Cheers to you, Sonya!

Serving:
2–2.5 quarts

Prep Time:
20 minutes

Ingredients

- 6-8 fresh lemons
- 2 cups sugar
- ½ cup fresh or frozen raspberries
- 6-8 cups water

Directions

1. Make simple syrup by combining 2 cups water and 2 cups sugar in a saucepan on the stove. Simmer on medium heat until sugar is fully dissolved. Set aside to cool to room temperature.
2. Juice 6-8 lemons (approximately 1 ½ cups juice) using a hand or electric juicer. Strain through a fine mesh strainer to remove seeds or pulp.
3. Heat ½ cup raspberries for 30 seconds to a minute in the microwave. Mash in fine mesh strainer over lemon juice until all raspberry juice runs through and you're left with thickened raspberry pulp.**
4. Mix simple syrup into lemon & raspberry juice. Add 4-6 cups of additional cold water until sweetness is to your preferred taste.
5. Garnish with lemon slices and/or fresh raspberries and/or mint leaves and chill.
6. Enjoy!

Variations

- Substitute any fresh fruit for raspberries. (Strawberries or blackberries would be especially good!)

Note:
**Keep raspberry pulp and use it to top pancakes/waffles, mix into other recipes, use on toast, etc.

Double Recipe (4-5 quarts)

- 12-16 fresh lemons
- 4 cups sugar
- 1 cup fresh or frozen raspberries
- 12-16 cups water

Single Serve (1 quart)

- 3-4 fresh lemons
- 1 cup sugar
- ¼ cup fresh or frozen raspberries
- 3-4 cups water

Beverages

Homemade Hot Chocolate

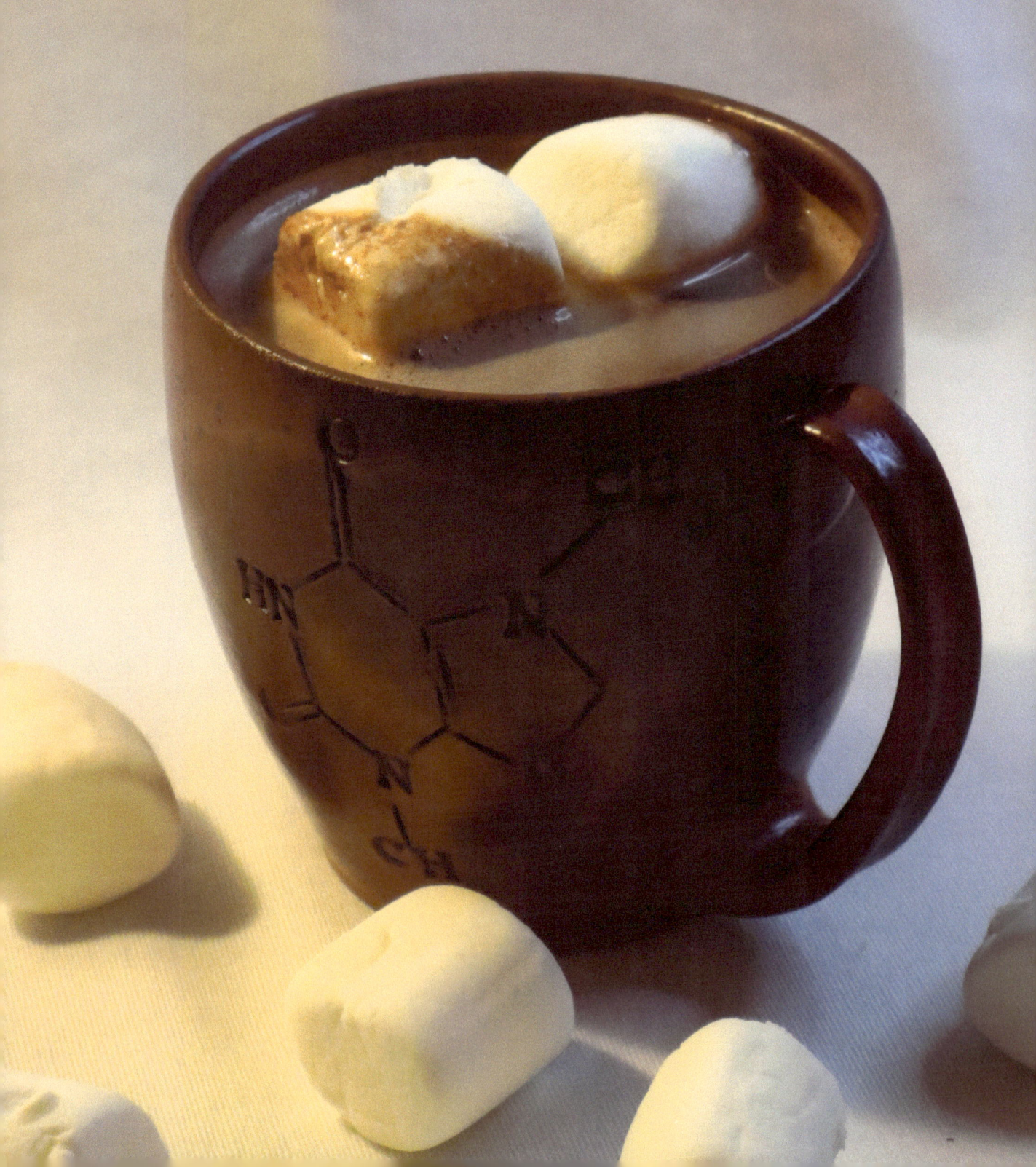

I am a hot chocolate fan. Any season, hot or cold, I'm up for hot chocolate and marshmallows. Some of my all time favorite memories with my best friend, Lisa, were spending hours sipping hot chocolate at the French Broad Chocolate Lounge in Asheville NC and having amazing, down-the-rabbit-hole random conversations. I miss her every day, but sipping this hot chocolate out of the mug she gave me always helps me feel connected to her. Chocolate is love. At least in my world.

Serving:
2 people

Prep Time:
10 minutes

Ingredients

- 20 oz milk
- ¾ cup chocolate chips
- Splash of vanilla

Directions

1. Heat milk and vanilla in a saucepan on medium heat.
2. Add chocolate chips, stirring frequently until completely melted.
3. Remove from heat and froth with milk frother or electric whisk for 30 seconds – 1 minute.
4. Pour into mugs, add whipped cream or marshmallows as desired and drink up!

Variations

- Can substitute non-dairy milk as desired.
- Add peppermint stick or cinnamon stick for added fun flavor.
- To make an adult beverage, add peppermint schnapps, Bailey's, etc.
- Use dark or semisweet or milk chocolate chips, depending on your preference.

Double Recipe (4 people)

- 3 ½ cups milk
- 1 ½ cups chocolate chips
- 1 tsp of vanilla

Single Serve (1 person)

- 10 oz milk
- ½ cup + 2 tbsp chocolate chips
- Splash of vanilla

Peanut Butter Hot Chocolate

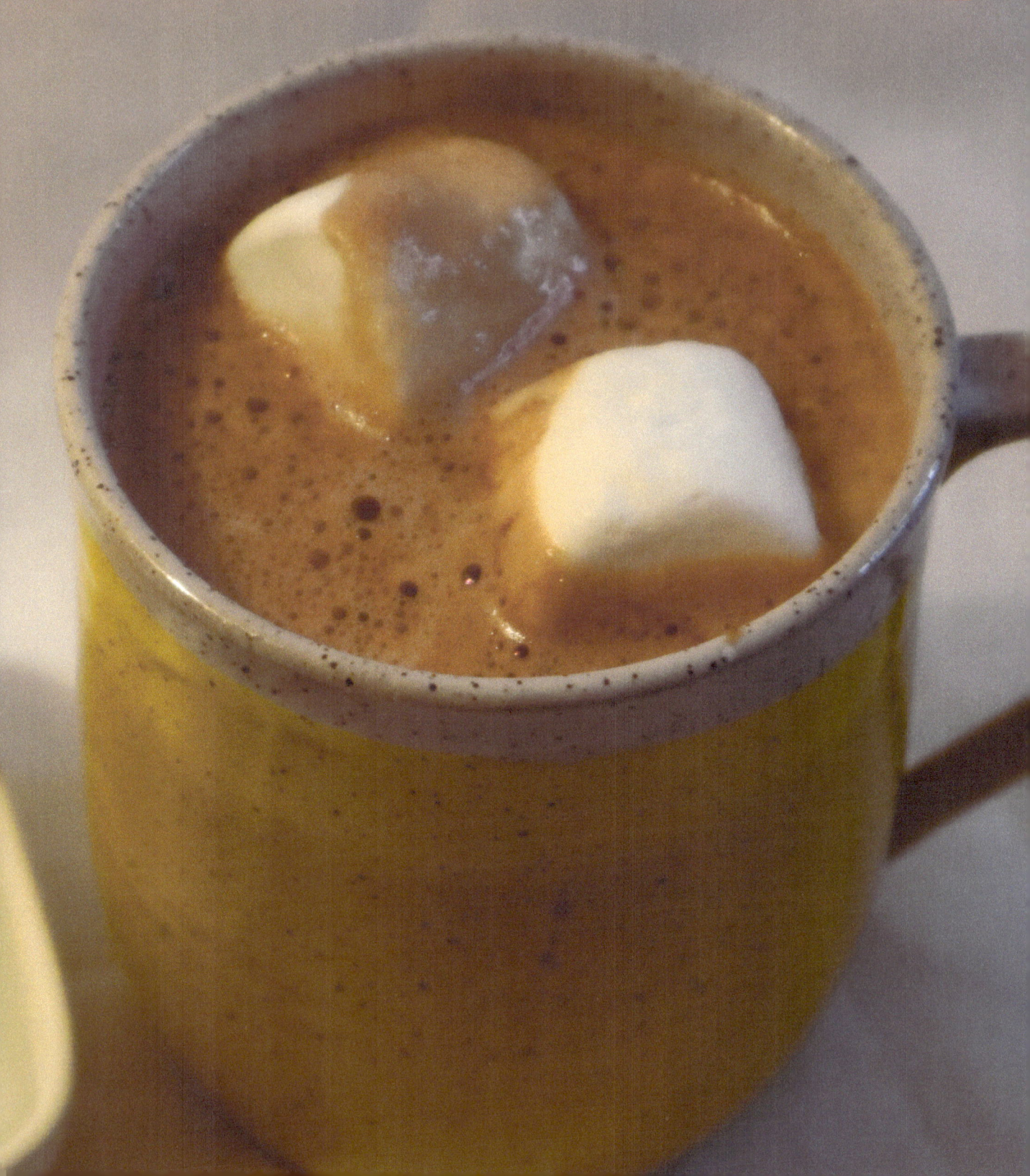

Nothing goes together better than chocolate and peanut butter! Rich, sweet, delicious flavor in a cup of soothing warmth for any chilly day. Savor every last glorious sip.

Serving:
2 people

Prep Time:
10 minutes

Ingredients

- 20 oz milk
- ½ cup chocolate chips
- ¼ cup peanut butter chips
- Splash of vanilla

Directions

1. Heat milk and vanilla in a saucepan on medium heat.
2. Add chocolate and peanut butter chips, stirring frequently until completely melted.
3. Remove from heat and froth with milk frother or electric whisk for 30 seconds – 1 minute.
4. Pour into mugs, add whipped cream or marshmallows as desired and drink up!

Variations

- Can substitute non-dairy milk as desired.
- Add peppermint stick or cinnamon stick for added fun flavor.
- Replace ¼ of the milk with heavy cream for extra creamy decadence.

Double Recipe (4 people)

- 3 ½ cups milk
- 1 cup chocolate chips
- ½ cup peanut butter chips
- 1 tsp vanilla

Single Serve (1 person)

- 10 oz milk
- ¼ cup chocolate chips
- 2 tbsp peanut butter chips
- Splash of vanilla

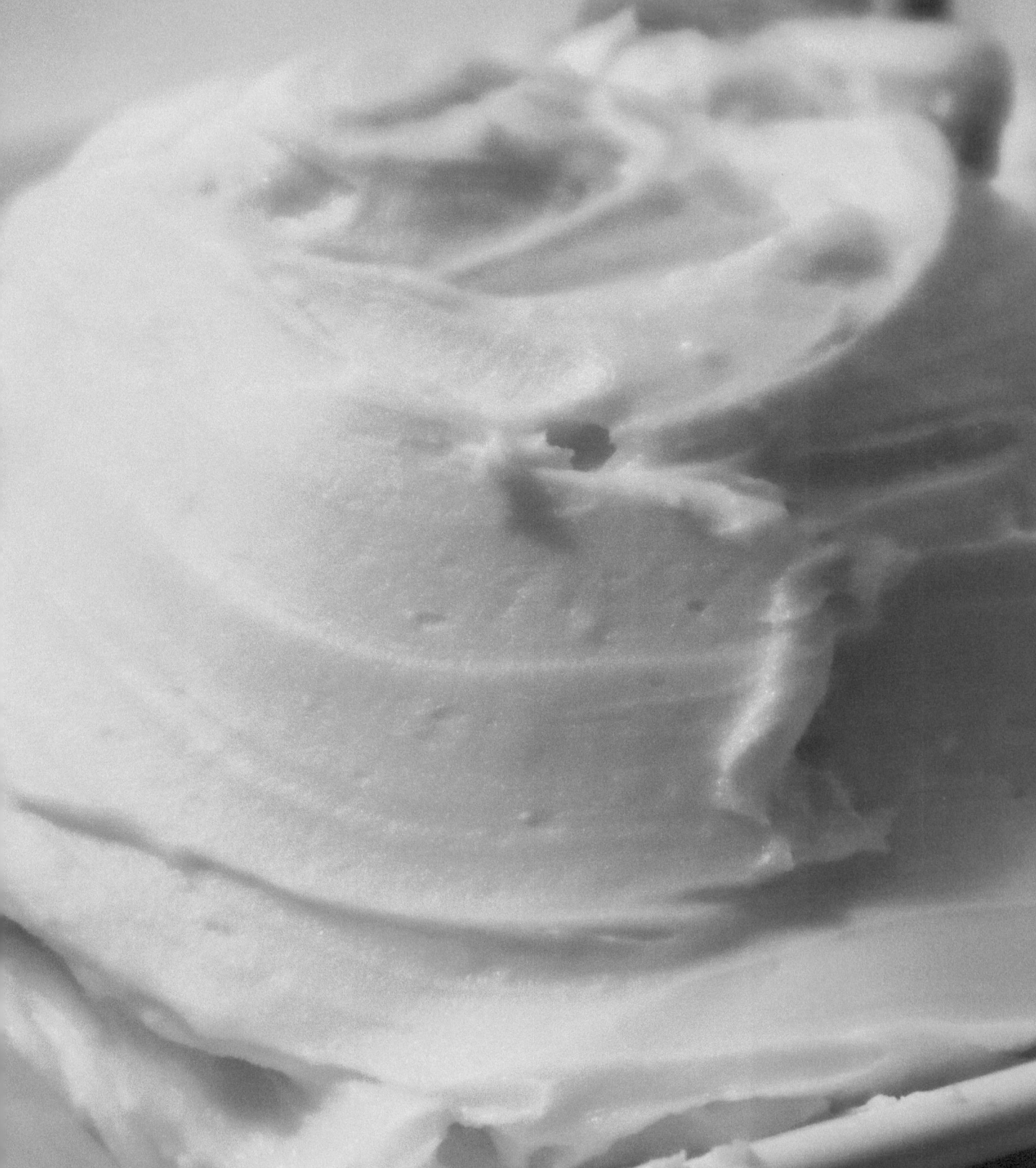

Serving:
9-inch cake

Prep Time:
10 minutes

Frostings & Fillings

Ingredients

- 8 tbsp softened butter (1 stick)
- 2 oz softened cream cheese
- 1 ½ cups powdered sugar
- 2 tsp vanilla

Directions

1. Beat butter and cream cheese together until light and fluffy (about 3-4 minutes).
2. Add powdered sugar and vanilla and beat until whipped (about 2 minutes).

Variations

- Add 2 tbsp of cocoa powder, raspberry/strawberry powder, peanut butter or other flavorings.
- Add food coloring.
- Mix sprinkles in for tie-dye effect.

> **Note:**
> Make dairy free: replace butter with vegan butter, omit cream cheese, and add enough vegan milk to get thickness or consistency you want.

Double Recipe
(two 9-inch cakes)

- 16 tbsp softened butter (2 sticks)
- 4 oz softened cream cheese
- 3 cups powdered sugar
- 4 tsp vanilla

Single Serve
(mini 4-inch cake)

- 4 tbsp softened butter (½ stick)
- 1 oz softened cream cheese
- ¾ cup powdered sugar
- 1 tsp vanilla

Royal Icing

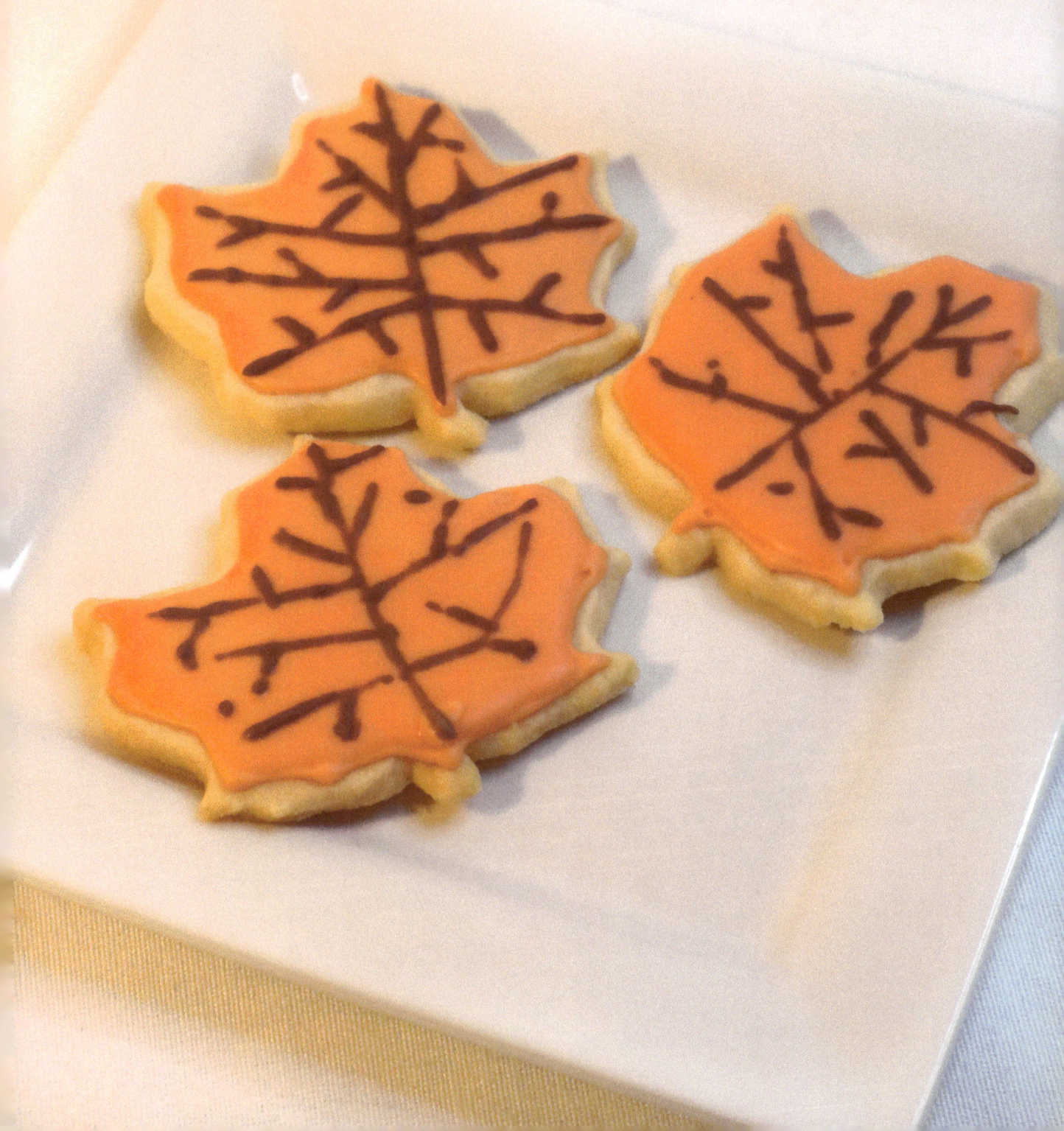

Serving:
3 cups

Prep Time:
5 minutes

Ingredients

- 4 cups powdered sugar
- 2 tbsp meringue powder
- ½ cup + 1–2 tbsp water, room temp
- 1 tsp vanilla
- Optional: food coloring

Directions

1. In a large bowl, beat all ingredients (except food coloring) together on high speed for 1–2 minutes, until icing drizzles down and smooths out within 5-10 seconds.
2. If too thick, add a little more water (very slowly). If too thin, add a little more powdered sugar.
3. Divide and color with food coloring as desired.

Variations

- Flavor with extracts as desired (peppermint, raspberry, lemon, etc.)

Note:

Will dry in about 2 hours at room temp, more quickly if placed in the fridge.

To keep from hardening while icing, cover unused portions of icing with a damp paper towel or put in an airtight container.

Double Recipe (6 cups)

- 8 cups powdered sugar
- 4 tbsp meringue powder
- 1 cup + 3-4 tbsp water, room temp
- 2 tsp vanilla
- Optional: food coloring

Single Serve (1½ cups)

- 2 cups powdered sugar
- 1 tbsp meringue powder
- ¼ cup + ½ to 1 tbsp water, room temp
- ½ tsp vanilla
- Optional: food coloring

Frostings & Fillings

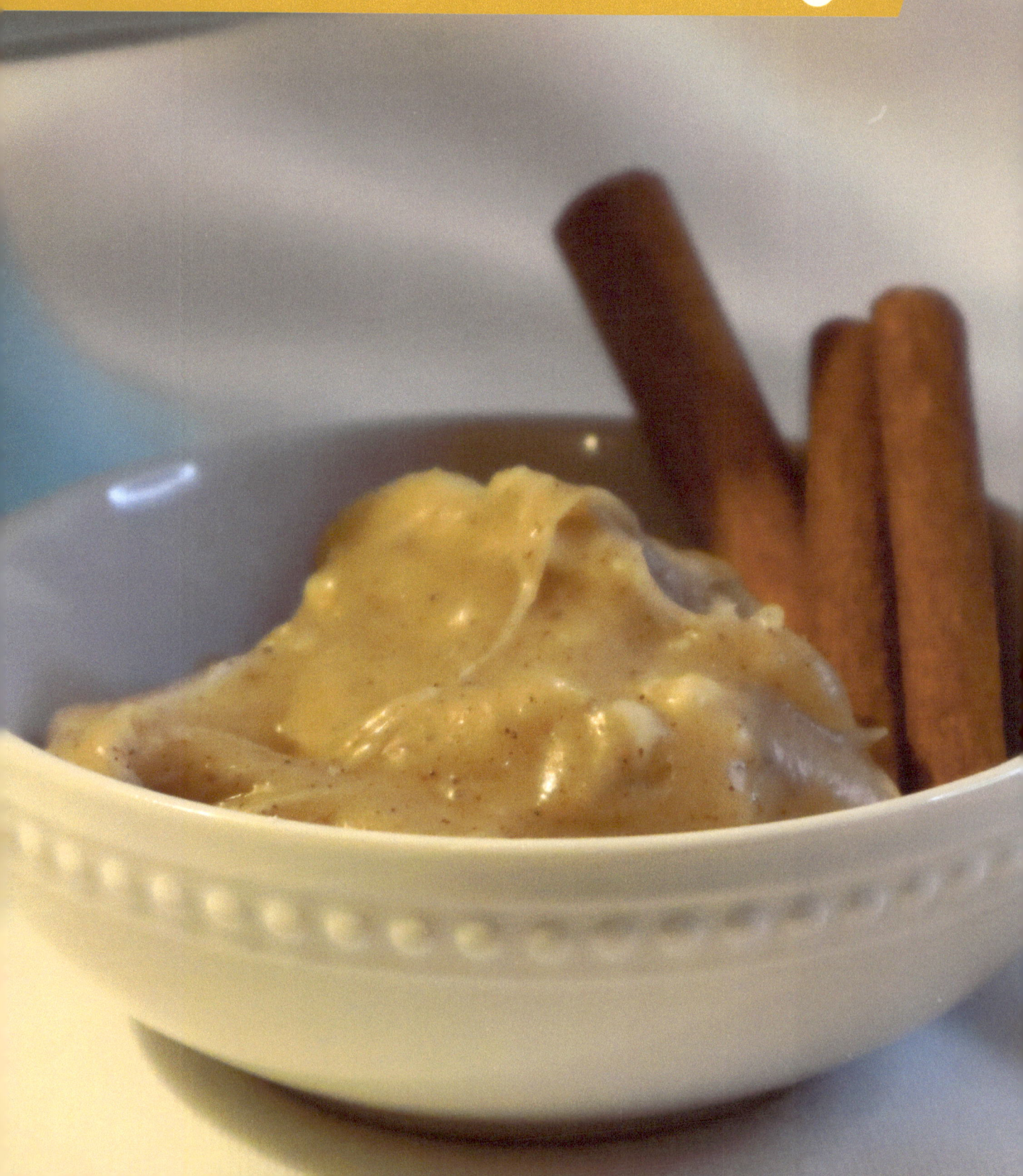

Cream Cheese Frosting

Serving:
12 cupcakes

Prep Time:
10 minutes

Ingredients

- ¼ cup softened butter
- 4 oz cream cheese, softened (brick-style)
- 1 tsp vanilla
- ⅛ tsp salt
- 2 cups powdered sugar

Directions

1. Cream butter and cream cheese until smooth and lump free.
2. Add vanilla and salt and mix well.
3. Gradually add powdered sugar until completely combined.
4. Frost completely cooled cake or cupcakes.

Variations (for regular size recipe)

- Chocolate: (¼ cup melted semi sweet chocolate.)
- Raspberry/strawberry: (Mix ¼ – ⅓ cup powdered freeze-dried fruit with powdered sugar.)
- Peanut Butter: (Add ⅓ cup creamy peanut butter.)

Note:

Do not freeze.

Can be stored in an airtight container for about a week.

Double Recipe (24 cupcakes)

- ½ cup softened butter
- 8 oz cream cheese, softened (brick-style)
- 2 tsp vanilla
- ¼ tsp salt
- 4 cups powdered sugar

Single Serve (6 cupcakes)

- 2 tbsp softened butter
- 2 oz cream cheese, softened (brick-style)
- ½ tsp vanilla
- Pinch of salt
- 1 cup powdered sugar

Frostings & Fillings

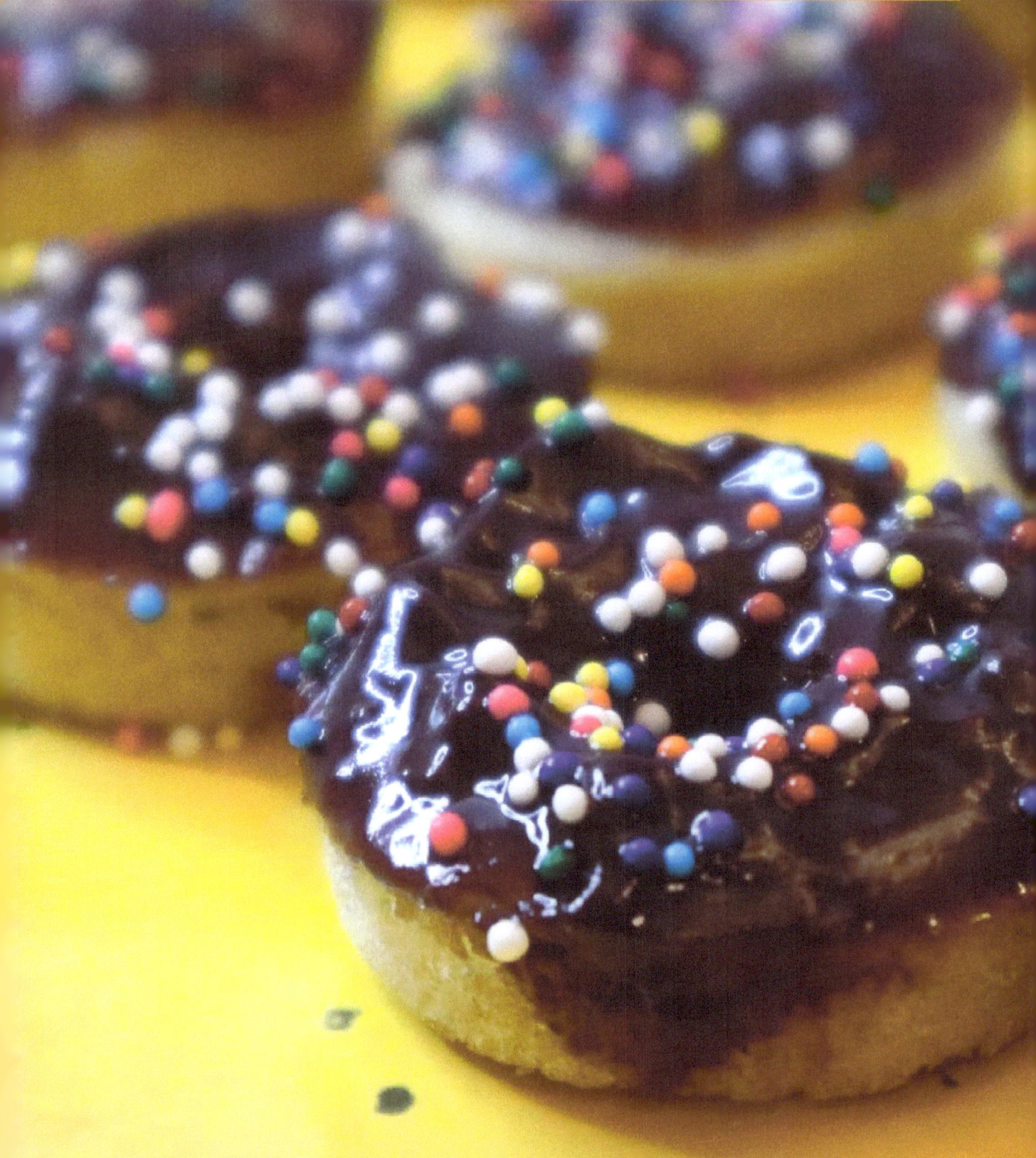

Dark Chocolate Ganache

Serving:
Approximately 1 cup

Prep Time:
10 minutes

Ingredients

- ¾ cup heavy cream
- 6 oz dark chocolate chips
- 2 tbsp butter, room temp

Directions

1. Heat heavy cream in a saucepan until just beginning to simmer.
2. Remove from heat and add chocolate chips. Let sit for a few minutes.
3. Whisk cream and chocolate together until smooth and shiny.
4. Add butter, a piece at a time and whisk well.
5. Use per recipe instructions.

Variations

- Can substitute milk or semisweet chocolate as desired.

Double Recipe
(Approximately 2 cups)

- 1 ½ cups heavy cream
- 12 oz dark chocolate chips
- 4 tbsp butter, room temp

Single Serve
(Approximately ½ cup)

- ¼ cup + 2 tbsp heavy cream
- 3 oz dark chocolate chips
- 1 tbsp butter, room temp

Frostings & Fillings

Chocolate Mousse

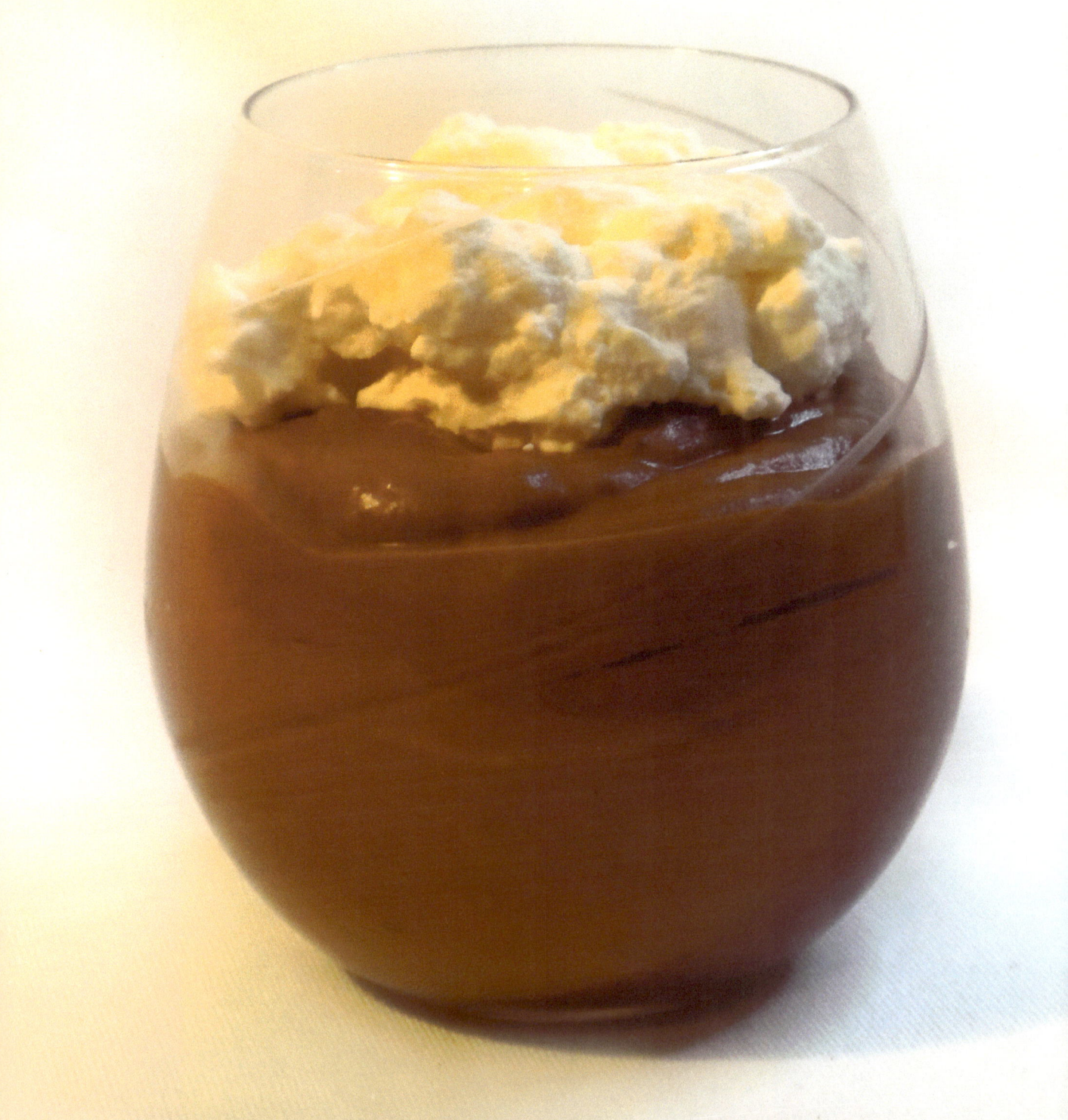

Serving:
1 ½ cups

Prep Time:
15 minutes

Ingredients

- 1 tsp + ⅛ tsp powdered gelatin
- 1 ½ tbsp water
- 9 ounces semisweet chocolate chips
- 1 ½ cups + ¾ cup heavy whipping cream, divided
- ¼ cup powdered sugar

Directions

1. In small bowl, sprinkle the gelatin over water, let stand for 5 minutes.
2. Place chocolate chips in medium bowl.
3. Heat ¾ cup of heavy cream until it comes to a full boil.
4. Add gelatin to heavy cream and whisk until dissolved.
5. Pour cream over chocolate chips and let sit for a minute.
6. Whisk until chocolate is melted and smooth. Set aside to cool about 5 minutes.
7. Whisk remaining heavy cream at high speed until it begins to thicken.
8. Add powdered sugar and whip until stiff peaks form.
9. Fold ⅓ whipped cream into chocolate mixture until well combined.
10. Add remaining whipped cream and fold.
11. Chill in the fridge for 2-3 hours to set.

Double Recipe (3 cups)

- 2 tsp + ¼ tsp powdered gelatin
- 3 tbsp water
- 18 ounces semisweet chocolate chips
- 3 cups + 1 ½ cups heavy whipping cream, divided
- ½ cup powdered sugar

Single Serve (¾ cup)

- ½ tsp + pinch powdered gelatin
- ¾ tbsp water
- 4 ½ ounces semisweet chocolate chips
- ¾ cup + ¼ cup and 2 tbsp heavy whipping cream, divided
- 2 tbsp powdered sugar

Frostings & Fillings

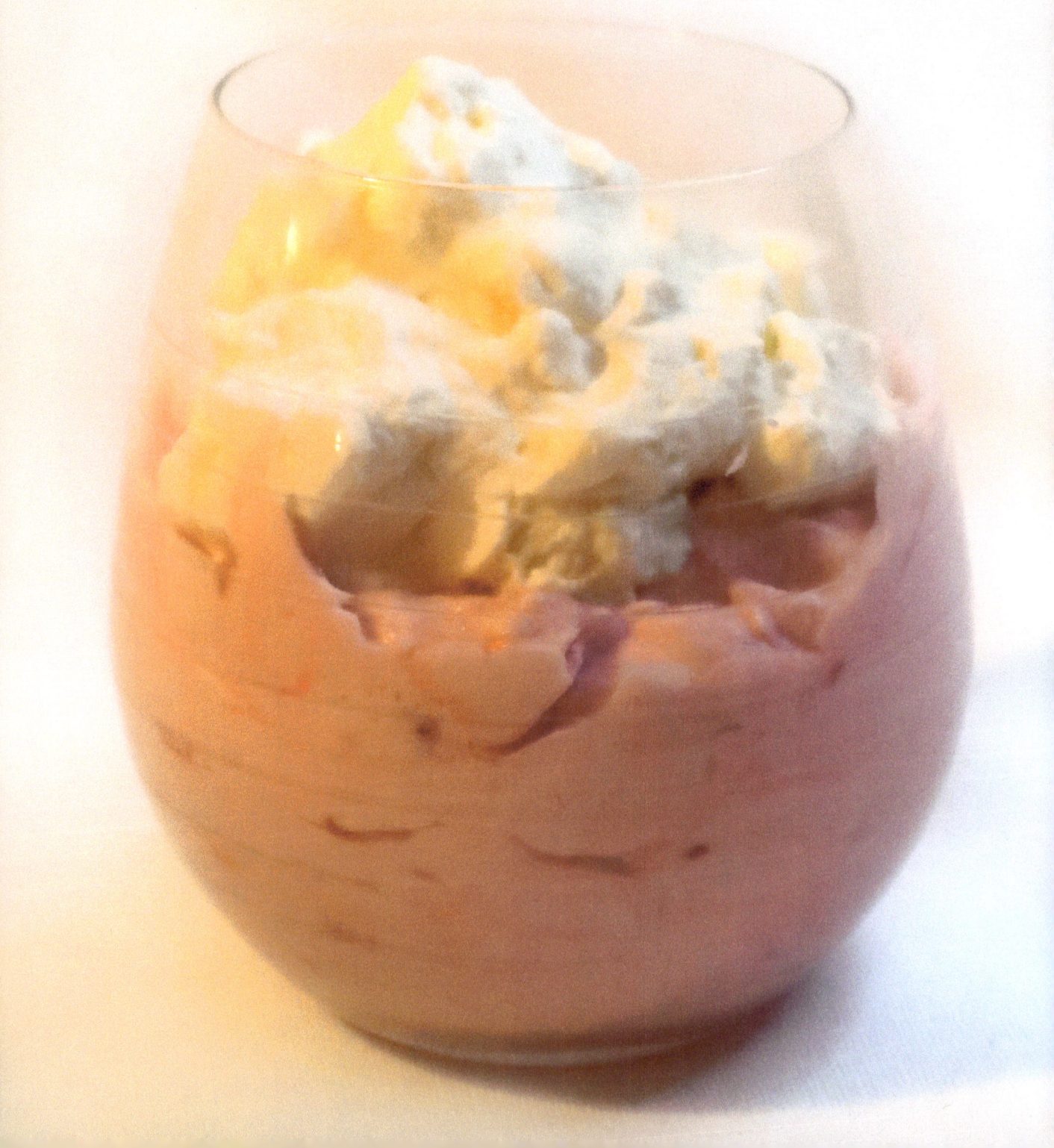

Serving:
1 ½ cups

Prep Time:
15 minutes

Ingredients

- ½ cup raspberries, frozen
- ¼ cup sugar
- 1 tbsp powdered sugar
- 1 ½ tbsp milk
- 1 ¼ cups whipping cream
- 1 ½ tsp powdered gelatin

Directions

1. In small bowl, sprinkle gelatin over water and let sit for 5 minutes.
2. Puree frozen raspberries.
3. Heat raspberry puree with sugar and milk on the stove until just beginning to simmer.
4. Whisk in gelatin until dissolved.
5. Strain through a fine mesh strainer to remove pulp and seeds.
6. Store pulp and seeds for use in other recipes.
7. Whip remaining heavy cream on high until it begins to thicken.
8. Add powdered sugar and whip until stiff peaks form.
9. Fold ⅓ whipped cream into raspberry juice until well combined.
10. Fold in remaining whipped cream.
11. Cool fridge for 2-3 hours to set.
12. Store in an airtight container in the fridge.

Variations

- Substitute strawberries, blueberries, blackberries, pineapple, etc. for raspberries.

Double Recipe (3 cups)

- 1 cup raspberries, frozen
- ½ cup sugar
- 2 tbsp powdered sugar
- 3 tbsp milk
- 2 ½ cups whipping cream
- 3 tsp powdered gelatin

Single Serve (¾ cup)

- ¼ cup raspberries, frozen
- 2 tbsp sugar
- ½ tbsp powdered sugar
- ¾ tbsp milk
- ½ cup + 2 tbsp whipping cream
- ¾ tsp powdered gelatin

Frostings & Fillings

Vanilla Pastry Cream

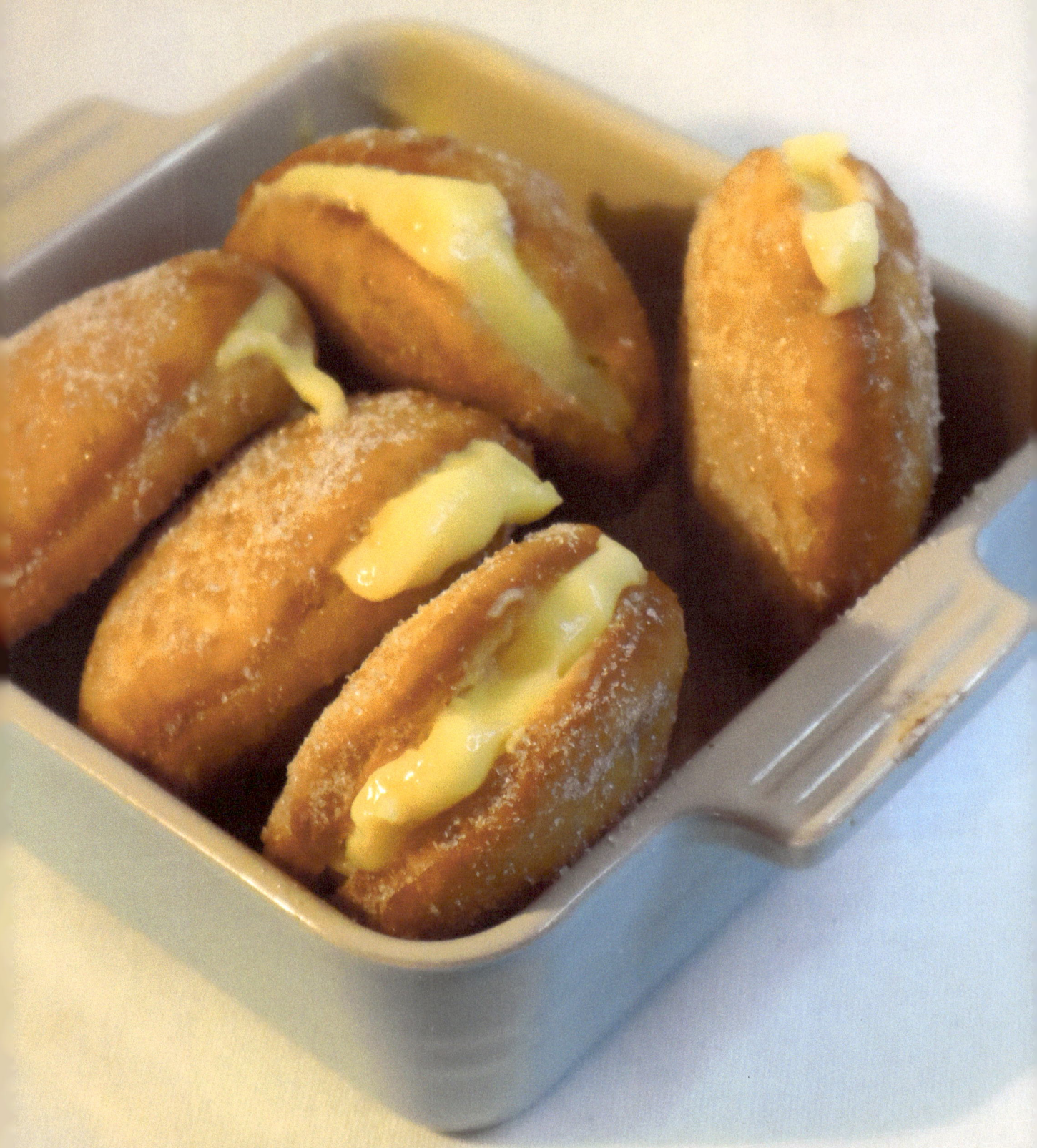

Serving:
1 cup

Prep Time:
5 minutes

Bake Time:
10 minutes

Frostings & Fillings

Ingredients

- 1 cup milk
- ½ tsp vanilla
- ⅛ tsp cornstarch
- 2 tbsp + 2 tsp sugar
- 1 egg yolk

Directions

1. Combine ¾ cup milk and vanilla in a medium saucepan. Cook over high heat until just beginning to simmer, stirring often. Remove from heat.
2. In a medium bowl, whisk remaining milk, egg yolk, sugar, and cornstarch.
3. While whisking vigorously, slowly pour hot milk into the egg mixture.
4. Return mixture to saucepan and cook over high heat, continuously whisking until it thickens and begins to boil.
5. Pass through a strainer and into a bowl.
6. Place plastic wrap directly on top of pastry cream to prevent a skin from forming.
7. Cool to room temperature, then place in the fridge for 2-3 hours to set. Whip before use.
8. Store in an airtight container in the fridge.

Note:
Do not freeze.

Double Recipe (2 cups)

- 2 cups milk
- 1 tsp vanilla
- ¼ tsp cornstarch
- ⅓ cup sugar
- 2 egg yolk

Single Serve (½ cup)

- ½ cup milk
- ¼ tsp vanilla
- Pinch of cornstarch
- 1 tbsp + 1 tsp sugar
- ½ egg yolk

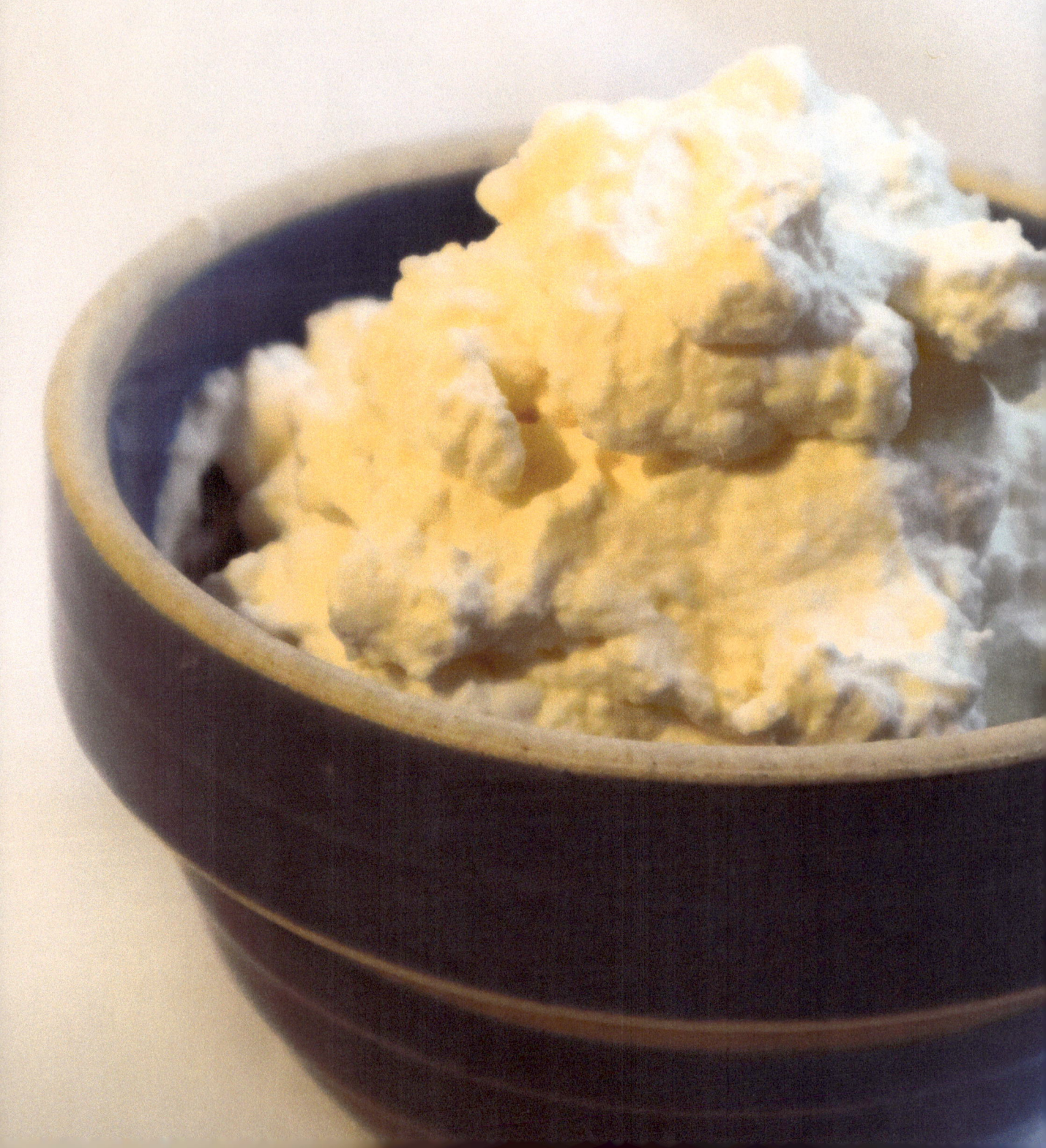

Whipped Cream

Serving:
3 cups

Prep Time:
10 minutes

Ingredients

- 1 cup cold heavy cream
- 2 tbsp powdered sugar
- 1 tsp vanilla

Directions

1. Whip heavy cream, sugar, and vanilla on medium-high speed until medium stiff peaks (about 3-4 minutes).

Variations

- Add 2-3 tbsp of cocoa or raspberry/strawberry powder for flavored whipped cream.

Note:

Can be kept in an airtight container in the fridge for up to 24 hours.

Add more or less powdered sugar to adjust sweetness.

Double Recipe (6 cups)

- 2 cups cold heavy cream
- ¼ cup powdered sugar
- 2 tsp vanilla

Single Serve (1½ cups)

- ½ cup cold heavy cream
- 1 tbsp powdered sugar
- ½ tsp vanilla

Frostings & Fillings

Baking Bloopers

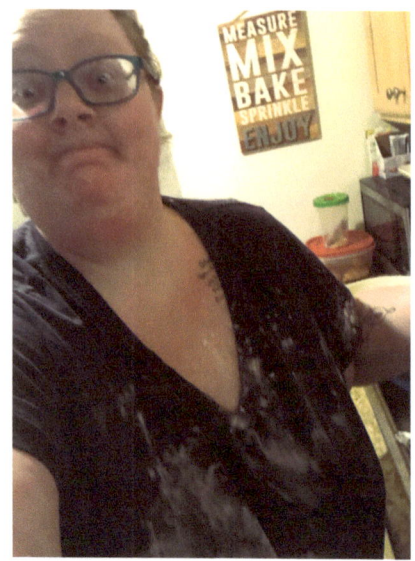

Why aprons are recommended

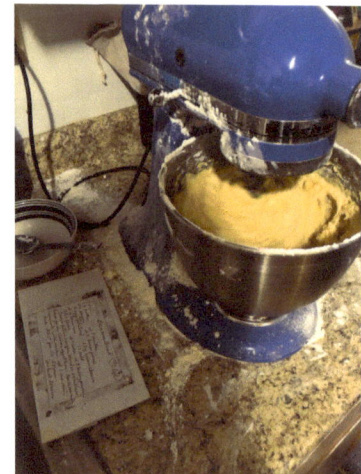

Flour mishaps

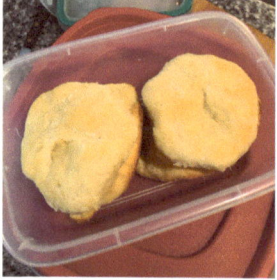

Tasty but flat biscuits

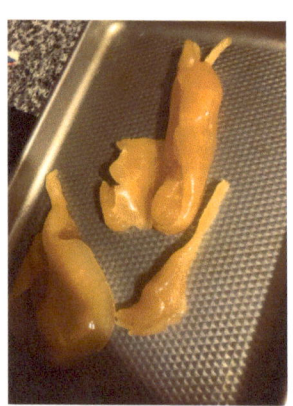

Taffy flop

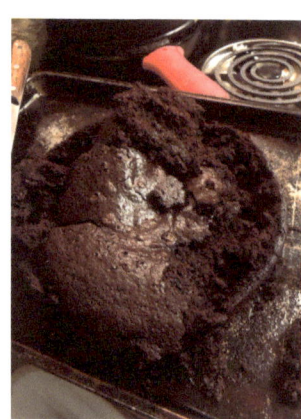

Cake layer cutting disasters

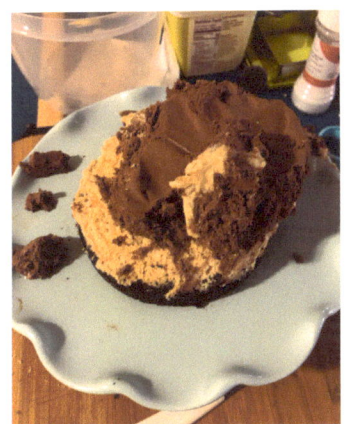
Ugh, cats underfoot

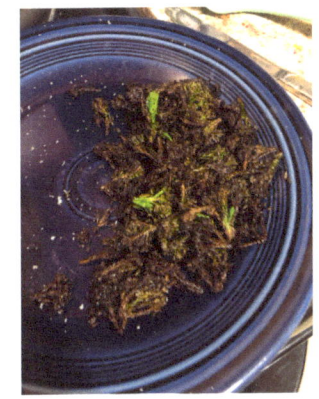
A little charcoal with your broccoli

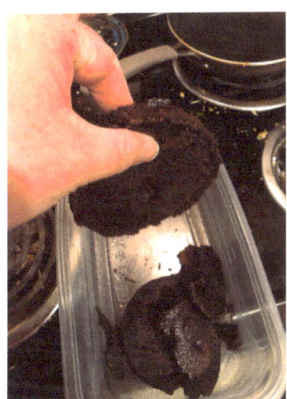
Too much water = rubbery cake

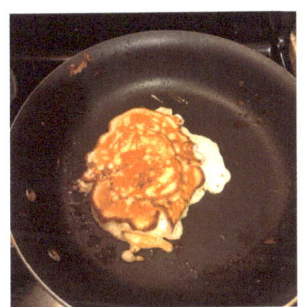
Tasty but ugly!

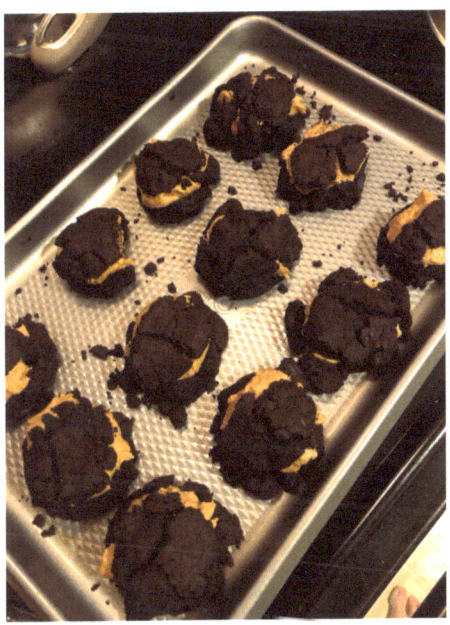
Cookie experiment gone awry

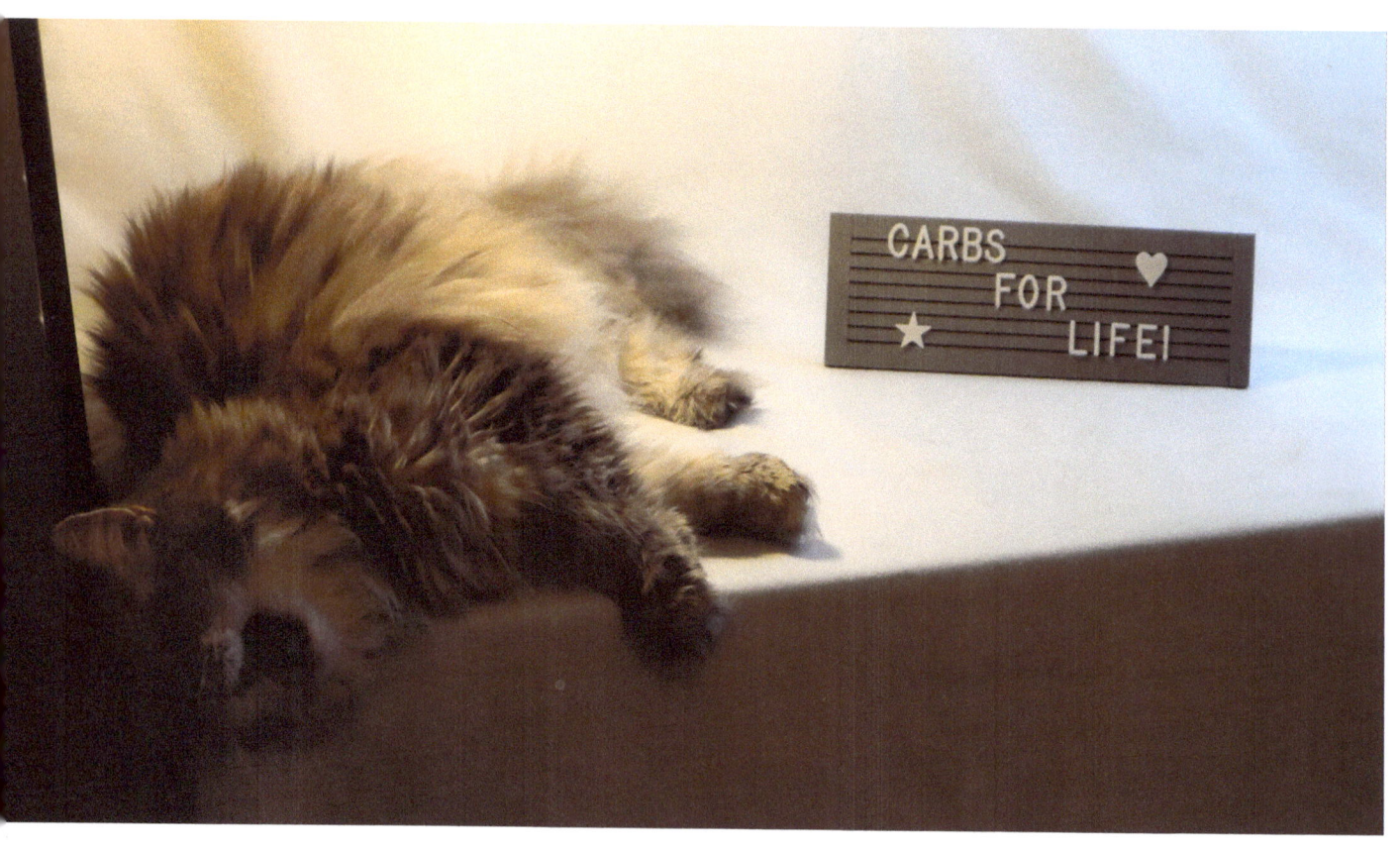

Gratitude & Thank You's

First, to my mom and her big silver bowl. Thanks for teaching me to make your chocolate chip cookies (and more!) all those years ago.

To my baking friends (especially Rachel)—for always talking about baking and food with me, for sharing tips and tricks, for listening to my ideas + giving me more of them, and everything else.

The Dabransky family, MK, Robin, and other local friends who helped consume all the excess baked goods that wouldn't fit in my freezer! And to friends around the country who helped eat up dozens of cookies and offered opinions on cookie experiments.

To my cats, Lillie and Luna, for patiently putting up with all the hours in the kitchen instead of snuggling with you. And for forgiving me for not sharing all the goodies. Sorry, floofs.

To the pandemic, you pain-in-the-ass global disaster that destroyed my social life and plans, but hey, I got a cookbook out of it. At least I ate well throughout.

To Sarah Hubbard, for the beautiful design work and making all this info transform into a real cookbook.

To Isora Lithgow, for the amazing and fun kitchen photo shoot!

And to everyone who gives these recipes a try—this was a lot of fun to make.
I hope you enjoy! Come share your favorites—IG: @long.emily

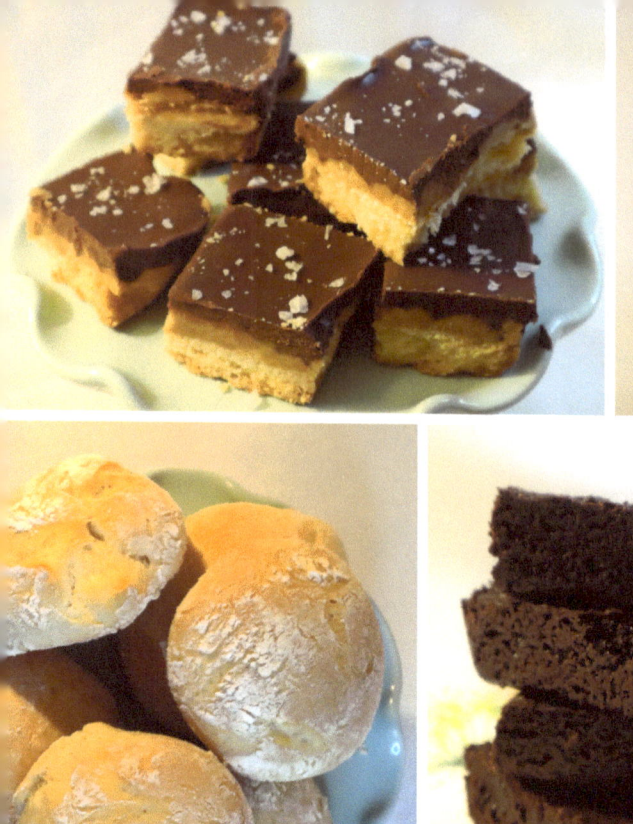
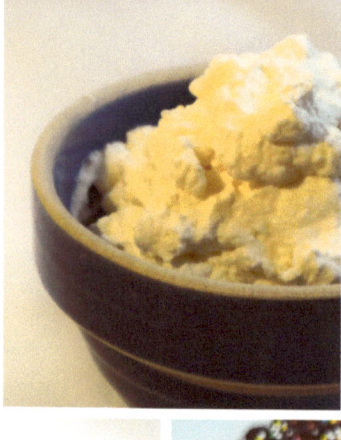
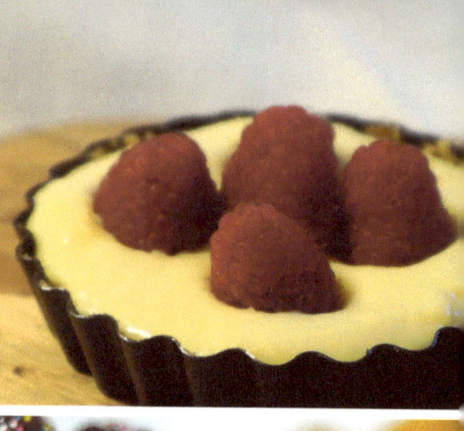
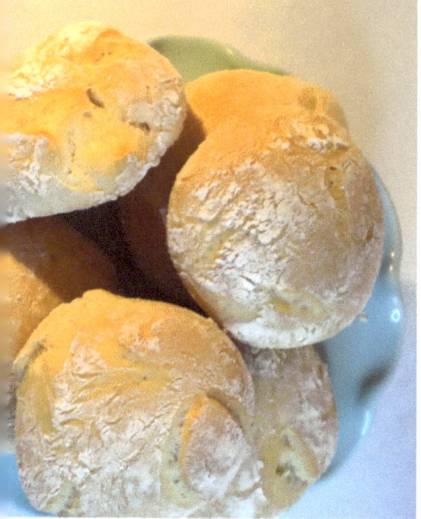
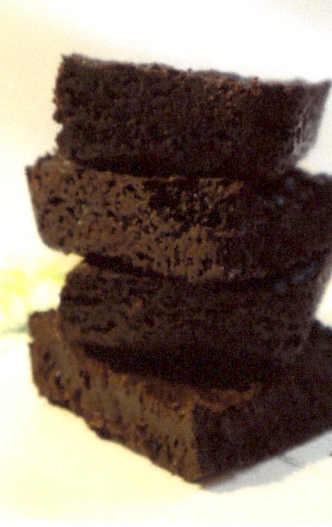
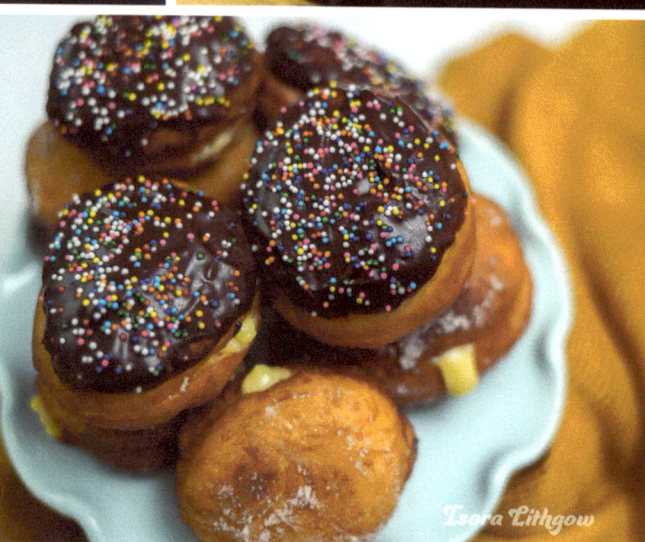
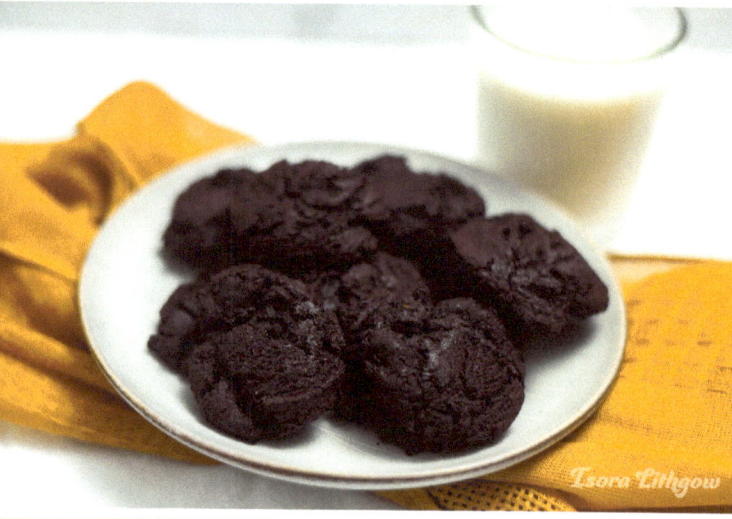
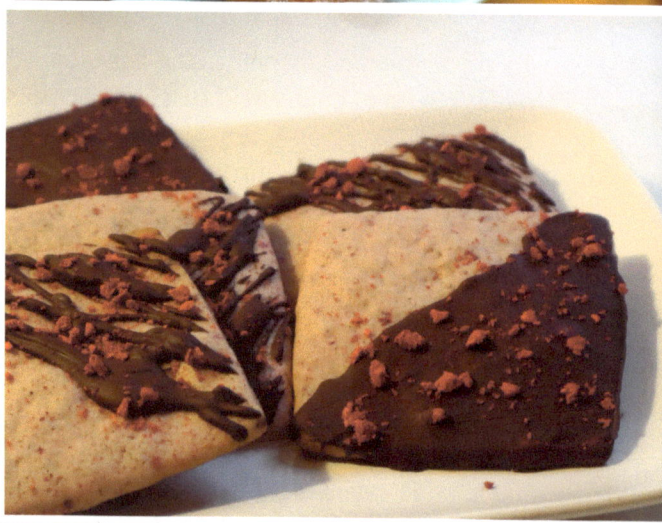
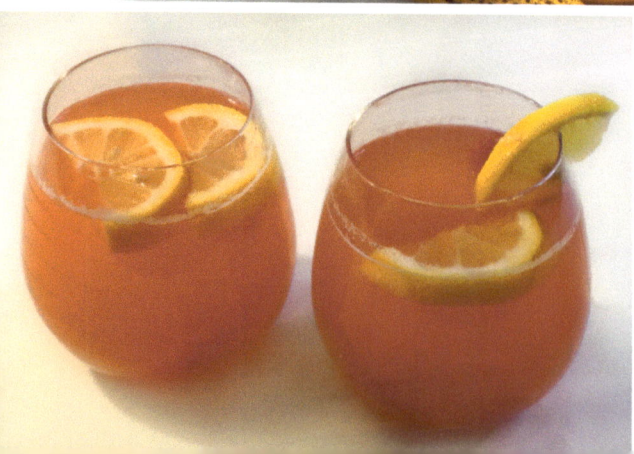
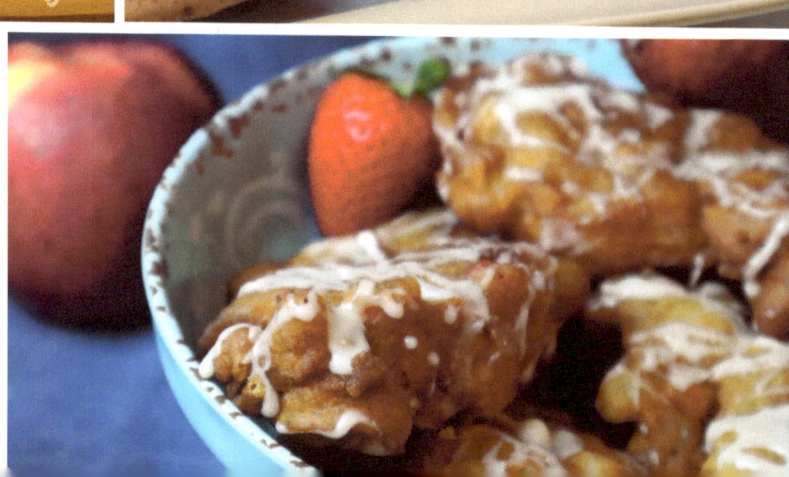

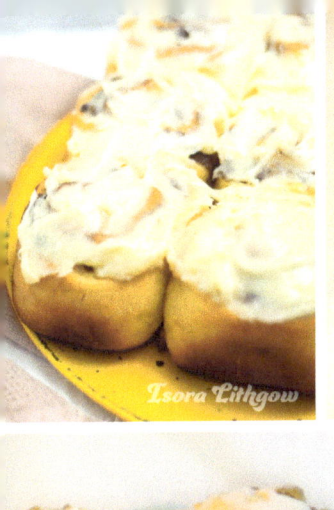
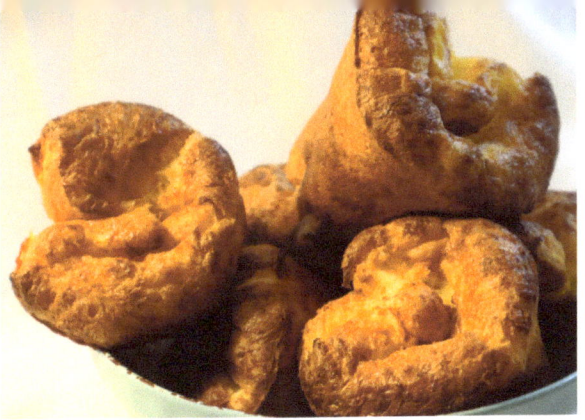
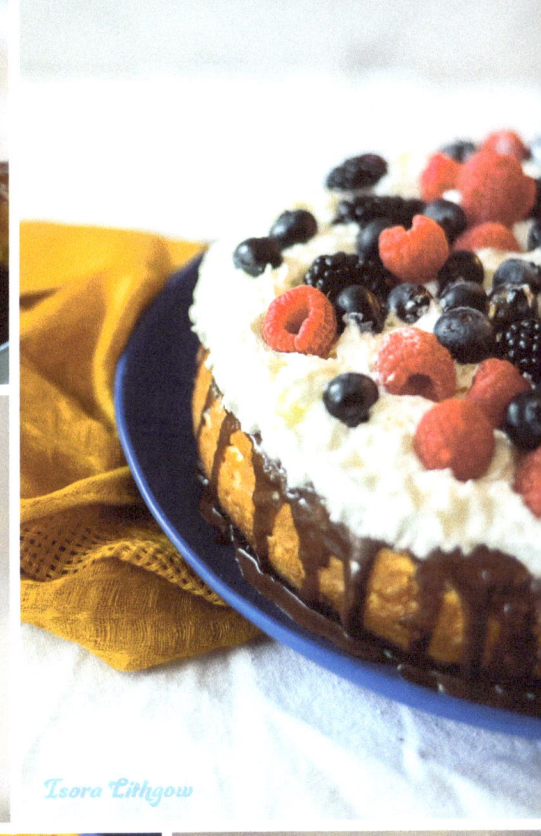
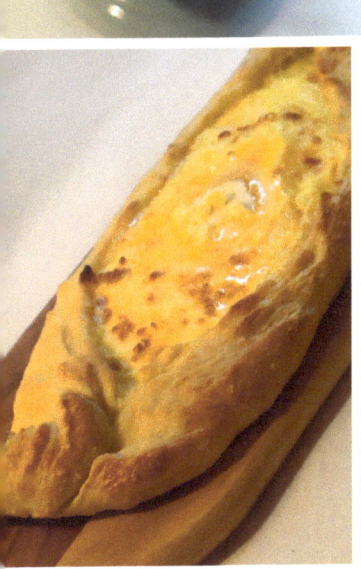
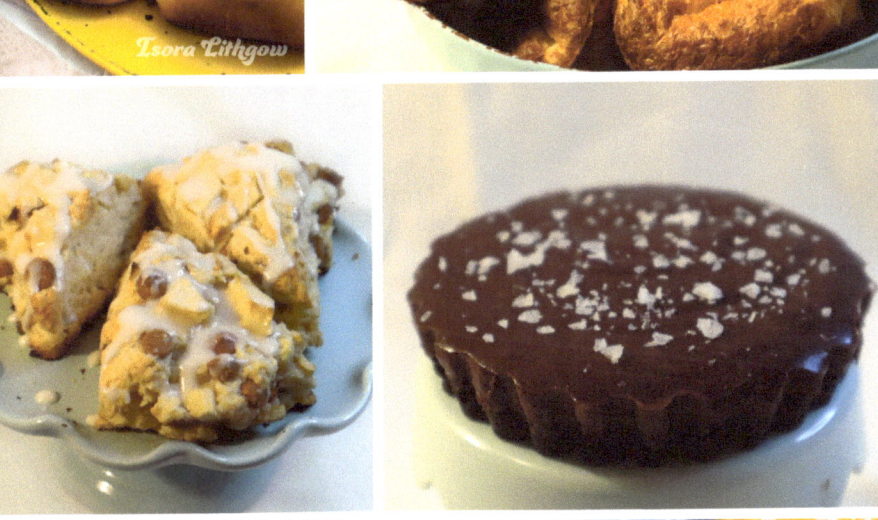
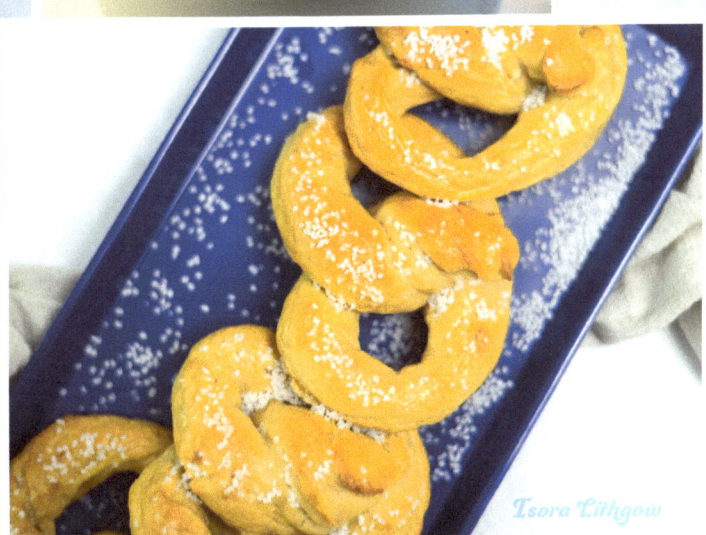
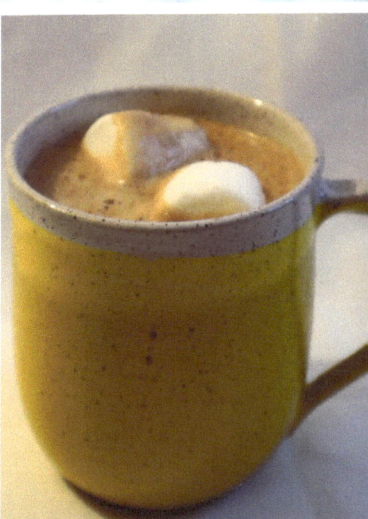
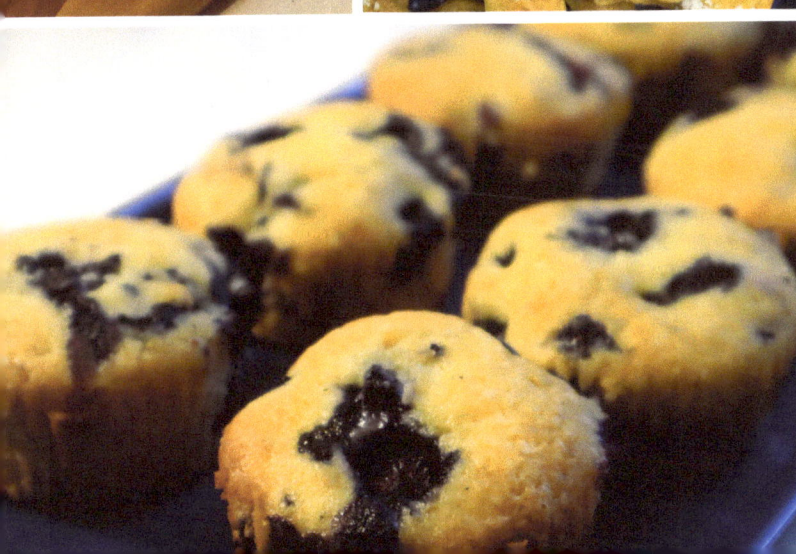
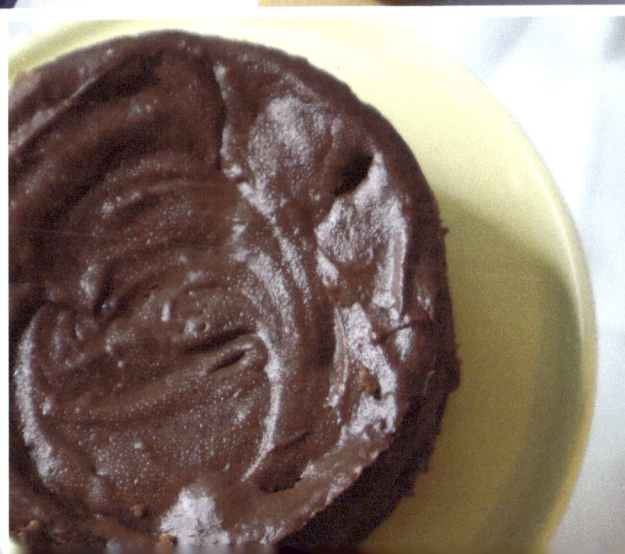

www.ingramcontent.com/pod-product-compliance
Lightning Source LLC
Chambersburg PA
CBHW041102070526
44583CB00002B/26